FAST-FOOD KIDS

CRITICAL PERSPECTIVES ON YOUTH

General Editors: Amy L. Best, Lorena Garcia, and Jessica K. Taft

This series aims to elaborate a set of theoretical and methodological tenets for a distinctive critical youth studies rooted in empirical inquiry. The series draws upon the following as some of the key theoretical elements of critical approaches: the socially constructed nature of childhood and adolescence over and against the universalizing and naturalizing propensities of early developmental theory; the centering of young people's social worlds and social locations as the starting point for analysis; exploration of how the meaning and experience of youth is shaped by other important axes of social difference, including but not limited to race, class, gender, place, nation, and sexuality; the recognition that youth's worlds are constituted through multiple processes, institutions, and discourses, and that central to understanding youth identity and experience is understanding social inequalities; engagement with the dynamics of global transformation in the experience of childhood and youth; and the relevance of these elements for policy and practice.

Books in the series:

Fast-Food Kids: French Fries, Lunch Lines, and Social Ties
Amy L. Best

Fast-Food Kids

French Fries, Lunch Lines, and Social Ties

Amy L. Best

NEW YORK UNIVERSITY PRESS
New York

NEW YORK UNIVERSITY PRESS
New York
www.nyupress.org

References to Internet websites (URLs) were accurate at the time of writing. Neither the author nor New York University Press is responsible for URLs that may have expired or changed since the manuscript was prepared.

ISBN: 978-1-4798-4270-4 (hardback)
ISBN: 978-1-4798-0232-6 (paperback)

For Library of Congress Cataloging-in-Publication data, please contact the Library of Congress.

New York University Press books are printed on acid-free paper, and their binding materials are chosen for strength and durability. We strive to use environmentally responsible suppliers and materials to the greatest extent possible in publishing our books.

Manufactured in the United States of America

10 9 8 7 6 5 4 3 2 1

Also available as an ebook

For my sister, Christine, and my daughters, Annie and Ella

CONTENTS

The topic of what kids eat and who is feeding them has generated an outpouring of interest in public and policy realms in recent years, triggering a substantial research and policy investment, as well as major grassroots efforts to improve young people's dietary health. We have seen lots of prescriptions for change. There is good reason to direct our energies to improving what young people eat and the circumstances that influence their diet, since we know eating habits formed in childhood, as well as access to nutrient-rich foods in childhood, have consequences for dietary health in adulthood. We know that a shockingly large number of young people in the United States do not meet the daily dietary guidelines set by the federal government for fruits, vegetables, and whole grains but instead consume large quantities of energy-dense, nutritionally poor processed foods. About 40 percent of American teens consume fast food every single day; teens more than any other age group report visiting fast-food restaurants for an afternoon snack; a large number of American families across income groups rely on fast foods to get dinner on the table.[1] We also know that some kids eat better than others. Children's dietary health is associated with poverty and inequality, both inseparable from a legacy of segregation and social indifference.

Without a doubt, what young people eat is influenced by the messages from the commercial food industry. Fast foods, usually cheap, processed foods, high in salt, fat, and sugar, are heavily marketed to youth; African American and Hispanic children are disproportionately targeted by commercial food markets. In 2012, fast-food restaurants placed six billion display ads on Facebook alone.[2] Yet as much as we know young people are inundated with messages promoting the value of cheap burgers and salty fries, soda and Doritos, we know much less about the social meanings young people give to food or the social contexts in which they consume it.

Understanding food's meaning as it is individually and collectively understood by kids as they eat at school, hang out at McDonald's, and head home for dinner at the end of the day has tremendous relevance for the way social researchers and advocates for food policy and behavioral change address young people's food consumption. This is why some interventions in dietary health succeed and others fall flat. If we want to effect positive change in what kids eat, we need to understand what food means for kids and how social context shapes that meaning. We need to understand not just the barriers to well-being that constrain young people but also their understandings of those barriers. And we need to understand the creative strategies kids use to live within them. This requires talking to young people and observing them in their everyday worlds.

Fast-Food Kids examines the food landscape where young people eat—at home, at school, and after school in fast-food settings like McDonald's, Taco Bell, Dairy Queen, and Chipotle—paying attention to the up-close scenes where kids eat and the broader backdrop of social change in American life that both constrains and makes possible specific ways of life. Such an inquiry carries some urgency at this historical moment as concerns grow over young people's food consumption and the place of commercial markets in their lives. While an increasing portion of young people's food consumption occurs outside the home, their food consumption within the home has become much more precarious. Despite this changing reality, we continue to associate food, especially food served to children, with the private sphere of home, even while millions of American families lack the means to provide nutrient-rich foods to their children, and others are prevented by the time burdens of our modern lives from doing so. At the same time, we are ambivalent about public provisioning of food in schools, and our ambivalence has real consequences for children, especially those who are poor. Unlike home-cooked food, which is cast as an object of love and longing, school food holds little sacred value; it is mass produced and stripped of its emotional value. The value we assign to the domestic sphere and the value we attach to public institutions help us to understand this ambivalence.

With these considerations in mind, *Fast-Food Kids* uses the tools of a type of sociological analysis focused on cultural and situational dynamics to understand what kids eat and why, shedding light on the important role social bonds, identity needs, memory and emotion, social distinction, and status play in the meaning and value assigned to food and ultimately young people's dietary behavior. Attention to the cultural economy of food brings into focus larger cultural narratives about dignity, care, status, and belonging that are entangled with youth's food consumption. Young people often desire commercial foods as an expression of their belonging in youth worlds. Food is an object of play in youth worlds, used for various social ends. Food is also part of a gift economy for teens, expressing both social status and friendship ties. These meanings, in turn, have significant influence on what kids eat and what they think about it. *Fast-Food Kids* casts light on this complex of meanings and calls for greater effort to understand social meaning and its context as we craft policies to promote dietary change and preserve our collective well-being.

ACKNOWLEDGMENTS

A great many people helped bring this book into being. At the center of my life are my two daughters and my husband, who are a continual source of love and happiness. Surrounding us is a terrifically loving and very large extended family with whom we have shared the most significant of life's moments. Their warmth, kindness, and generosity of spirit are sustaining. I appreciate the support I received from George Mason University, in particular the College of Humanities and Social Sciences, where I have found colleagues across departments with whom I feel a deep kinship and shared sense of purpose. The Department of Sociology and Anthropology at George Mason University is my intellectual home. Here I have a found a wonderful set of colleagues who have provided useful comment and steadfast support from this project's beginning. I feel lucky to belong to a group of social scientists who are as interested as they are interesting. As I began this project, our department launched a PhD program committed to public sociology. I served as its first director, bringing me into regular contact with a large number of intellectually engaged students, to whom I feel a debt of gratitude for their energy, curiosity, and spirit of possibility. I hope they have learned as much from me as I from them. Several students have been particularly instrumental in the progression of this project. Caroline Pendry and Nicole Hendert assisted with conducting interviews. Katie Kerstetter and J. L. Johnson also assisted with data collection for a broader food project that informs (though it extends well beyond) this book. A special thanks to the good folks at Arcadia's Center for Sustainable Food and Agriculture, with whom I have worked and from whom I have learned much; the two food directors at the schools I studied who gave of their time for this project; and my professors, whose teachings I bring with me to every project. The reviewers for this project provided excellent and helpful comment, as did many sociologists along the way. Finally, I am grateful to the editorial team at NYU Press, which has helped bring this book and others to print. Ilene Kalish has been my editor since I began writing and is an editor like no other.

I dedicate this book to my sister, Christine, who is a creative force for change and has demanded nothing less than a healthier future for us all, and to my daughters, Ella and Annie, for their uncommon goodness.

Introduction

Fast-Food Kids

In early fall of 2008, just as the school year has begun, I sit on a sunny Sunday afternoon at Baskin-Robbins, one of the many commercial food spots I have visited over the last several years, trying to understand how food figures in young people's daily lives. I watch as three high school girls walk to the shop's counter. Each is in athletic sweats sporting their high school logo, wearing traces of eyeliner and their long hair in that disheveled top bun I have come to associate with suburban girls who are into sports. One of the girls softly sings a current pop song. She has a beautiful voice and she sings to herself, playing with the melody, while the other two exchange small talk with giggles interspersed. They order a large sundae with three scoops, all chocolate, dripping with caramel and topped with whipped cream, to be shared among them, and I watch as a young woman appearing to be in her late teens prepares the sundae behind the counter. She is one of the few teen workers I have seen stand behind any fast-food counter in the five years I spent collecting data for this project. Most of the commercial fast-food workers at Panera, Chipotle, Baja Fresh, McDonald's, or Taco Bell in this area are immigrant adults, brown and accented, though many are in their early twenties.[1] (I learned later that this young worker's parents, immigrants from Korea, own the franchise, where the whole family works.)

One of the girls hands a carefully folded ten dollar bill to the girl behind the counter, who smiles as she returns her change and hands over the sundae, which is received with a polite "thanks," and the three girls find a seat at a small table to share the large ice cream sundae. All three sit lounge style, one girl with bent knee cradled against the edge of the table, another slouched in her seat with her legs extending forward toward the floor, her sloping back resting against her chair. Their talk is full of laughter, with giggles interjected between words as each clamors to speak over the other in fits and starts, all the while eating this single sundae. I hear one girl say, "I'm so full, so full!" and another chimes in, "Oh my god, look at my stomach!" A moment later the same round of comments is offered again —"I'm so full"; "Seriously, look at my stomach, it's bigger"—laughter bursting from the group, spilling over to where I sit two tables away. They seem simultaneously aware of and indifferent to the activity of others around them. Just then, one of the girls lets out a resounding burp. She giggles. Our eyes meet as she and I both glance in each other's direction. She offers, "Sorry," and I respond with a slight smile, "Quite alright." Our eyes break away and she returns to her friends as though I am no longer there and remarks to them that people think she is a trucker. They laugh at the apparent contradiction since she looks nothing like a typical trucker, and their talk resumes about the world of school, parents, friendship drama, and how some guy commented to some girl that she looked good in the jeans she was wearing. It is hard to miss the obvious pleasure these girls experience, reveling in this moment of what sociologist Randall Collins would likely characterize as "emotional entrainment," a cosmic bubbling up of girl energy as they play with gender boundaries and the feminine scripts that guide girls to adulthood, but also rein them in.[2] Theirs is a public act performed for me, for each other, and for anyone else who may care to take notice. And it serves multiple ends all in one fell swoop. Their performance helps to constitute them as a friendship group; it transforms this ordinary encounter into play; and it enables them to lay claim to this public space.[3]

And as tasty as that sundae may be, the ice cream's value, shared among them, is as a resource used for different conversational and social ends. This sundae's meaning lies in the extent to which it enables these girls to construct a social encounter and define the situation as a form of play that is central to the public display of youth culture and youth identity.[4] Anthropologist Mimi Nichter regards this type of talk as speech performance, which serves to provide freedom for girls, preempting scrutiny from other girls and serving to build rapport.[5]

Young people play with food all the time. They throw it—sometimes in an effort to thwart disclosure of an embarrassing tale told by a friend; they hold it over each other's heads as a kind of symbolic ransom or quid pro quo (You can have this piece of gum, if you help me with my homework); and they render strange the conventions and norms that govern how we "decipher a meal," to borrow a phrase from the anthropologist Mary Douglas. They reverse the order of foods—ice cream and cookies first, sandwich second. They consume obscene quantities in short order during food contests (sixty-four ounces of Yoo-hoo in sixty seconds, thirty White Castle burgers in a single sitting), which are popular among teenage boys.[6] These contests are then often posted to YouTube for the world to witness. Young people push the envelope with and through food and also play with food simply to pass the time. They actively invert accepted food categories and the appropriate time of day to eat them—spaghetti, moo shu pork, or pizza for breakfast— and proudly detail to friends their various food transgressions. What we eat and when we eat it are bounded by social rules that reflect our collective efforts to create and maintain a semblance of order out of the slices of activity that comprise our everyday worlds.[7] While very young children are learning and interpreting these social rules, older youth test them. Mary Douglas makes the point that these cultural categories are bound to and reflective of a moral ordering of objects that preserves hierarchical arrangements in groups and solidifies group membership and boundaries. Indeed, most of these categories find their origins in adult worlds, rising usually from the middle class. Thus, to play with these categories is to engage with an entire complex of social meanings that distinguish childhood from adulthood. Food is often about play for young people, used for strategic ends in a complex peer system of exchange and gift giving. Food is a social object through which social identities are conceived, tried on, and solidified (think about vegans) and with which youth display, sometimes in dramatic fashion, claims of belonging to age-based groups as well as demonstrate their proficiency in deciphering the cultural signs that mark the distance between youth and adult worlds. Food is thus a key cultural object in youth worlds, in large part because of the social ends food fulfills as gift, identity marker, and object of play.

Yet as much as food provides endless opportunity for play for youth, food is also bundled up with a broader set of economic and social relations that structure the everyday landscape of modern life, often providing context for the specific form play takes. Most food consumed today in what we now call the Global North is bought, despite a small but growing interest in homesteading, the revival of canning, and urban small-plot farming. Money is exchanged and food has been prepared and processed outside the home as part of what Anthony Winson refers to as "the industrial diet," comprised of foods that are mass produced by a small number of food-industry players into edible commodities that are highly processed, aggressively marketed, and nutritionally limited, especially when compared with whole foods. Contradictory forces of change at large-scale levels have reorganized food and its production, distribution, and consumption in profound ways in the last century.[8] While helping to reduce food shortages in the Western world, for instance, the rise of industrial agriculture has failed to improve nutritional health and food security and instead has spurred a new set of health risks with substantial global reach. The dynamics of food scarcity and food abundance, under-nutrition and over-nutrition, that mark today's food landscape express deepening economic inequalities locally and globally and are grafted along complex gender, national, class, ethno-racial, and spatial lines.[9] The dominance of industrial agriculture has also given rise to a global food movement calling for wholesale change to what many regard as a fundamentally broken and unsustainable food system, bad for our health and the environment. This movement for food reform is at once a movement to create equal food access for all and reduce food insecurity and at the same time a movement to reclaim the symbolic and cultural import of food, and thus it is motivated by moral considerations alongside economic ones.

Anthropologist Mary Douglas once described eating as "a field of action," a fitting characterization given the powerful symbolic resonance of food on the one hand, and its political-economic dimensions on the other.[10] Eating is both an economic and a cultural activity, part of a complex system of exchange in which food can be both commodity and gift, what the anthropologist Nicolas Thomas has called "entangled objects." In a strictly market-driven economic calculus, food is a commodity, not a gift. But of course, food does not simply have economic value. Other systems of value, what the anthropologist Fred Myers calls "regimes of value production," also organize the meaning of food, helping to explain why we eat some foods rather than others and how food fits into our social relations in a market-based economy.[11] As part of a gift economy, the exchange of food expresses and affirms group membership as well as boundaries of exclusion, communicating meaning about reciprocity, social obligation, and care.[12] As the anthropologist Arun Appadurai argues in *The Social Life of Things*, "a commodity is a thoroughly socialized thing."[13] As part of a gift economy in a market-based society, food exists within multiple spheres of exchange.

Food dwells in the realm of symbolic meaning, representing social distinction and inequality on the one hand, and belonging, intimacy, and care on the other—that is, the core dimensions of our collective life. Food consumption is tied to distinct taste communities, with each having different value commitments.[14] Today, in the Global North, our food choices are as likely to be determined by our aesthetic and moral sensibilities as by individual preference. (Consider, for instance, how ethical consumption of such food items as fair-trade coffee and chocolate serves as a means to project a moral self.)[15] Our ethnic selves are realized through food preparation and food consumption; feminine identities materialize through the provisioning and serving of meals for others on the one hand and the denial of food for self on the other.[16] Bound by and filtered through gender, race, and other cultural schema, food is used to classify and determine group boundaries. Groups of all types are sorted through food.[17] Again and again, kids remind me of this fact. I remember one afternoon when I first began this project, sitting at a McDonald's observing a group of kids munching french fries and sipping on twenty-four-ounce sodas after school. A mixed-race group of boys and girls sat across from me at two adjoining tables. Amid chatter about food kids have at home, one white girl with two long braids stretching to the middle of her back announced, "I have Kool-Aid at my house," to which a black boy, also at the table, quickly declared with wry incredulity, "You're not black." The group collapsed in laughter. Here Kool-Aid, an artifact of consumer culture that reached its heyday in the 1970s, is imagined in terms of racial belonging and membership. This was neither the first nor the last time I heard comments of this type. Instead racial, class, and gender constructs were fundamental to youth's engagement with food.

This central tension between food as material object and food as symbol organizes the core set of concerns examined in this book. *Fast-Food Kids* is an ethnography about food in the lives of American youth and the places where they eat. I hope to show how the entanglements of class, social context, and cultural meaning shape the ways youth relate to food as both symbol and material object, as both public and private good, while also accounting for the set of broader economic and political forces that have reshaped the current food landscape where young people eat. Looking at contemporary food practices—from family dinners with extended kin to solitary snacking in front of the screen, from take-home Chinese on Fridays to the drive-through for Taco Bell's breakfast burrito on Mondays, from school lunch to McDonald's fries after school—provides an opportunity to see the different types of relationships youth forge with food and food markets.

What Kids Eat and Why

In the last decade, the issue of what kids eat and who's feeding them has sparked an outpouring of public and policy discussion as increasing attention has been given to childhood obesity, a widespread phenomenon recognized by many from the world of public health as a global crisis in its own right.[18] The Robert Wood Johnson Foundation reports that obesity rates for children between the ages of six and eleven have quadrupled in the last half-century. Over twenty-three million children and teenagers are either obese or overweight.[19] The CDC (Centers for Disease Control) estimates that one in three American children is either overweight or obese—a number that is disproportionately higher for children living in concentrated poverty.[20] Though the CDC recently reported optimistically a small but significant downward trend in the prevalence of obesity among low-income, preschool-age children and the Robert Wood Johnson Foundation has reported modest decline across age groups in communities where comprehensive action to lower obesity rates among children has been taken, enduring inequalities in communities, schools, and homes have long structured young people's access to different types of food, shaping life chances, well-being, and a host of health outcomes.[21]

Young people as food consumers are now key figures in public health debates as schools and community health activists struggle to find creative ways to offset the tide of weight gain among our youngest children and, in some cases, work to create a platform to redress community-based social inequalities. Consider, for instance, First Lady Michelle

Obama's Let's Move campaign, spearheaded in 2008 to tackle childhood obesity, and federal and municipal policy reforms such as the 2010 D.C. Healthy Schools Act and the Healthy, Hunger-Free Kids Act of 2010. Designed to promote improved health and well-being through diet, all of these programs have helped to usher in change in public schools, though their long-term impact remains unclear. As a nation weighs in on the meaning of youth's food consumption and crafts policy and practice to transform what young people eat in an effort to stave off a host of diet-related health risks, it is important that we understand the social meaning young people themselves assign to food, and the cultural systems of value that organize those meanings. A core aim for this project, then, is to bring the tools of cultural analysis to bear on a topic that has captivated interest on the policy and grassroots levels. Policy work and practical interventions to increase access to and consumption of healthy foods have not focused enough on the collective meaning formed around food nor the schemes of value that organize those meanings. For example, while food is part of a complex system of gift exchange through which group boundaries are formed among youth peer groups, little policy attention has been given to how this matters to young people's food choices. Without attention to these considerations, health policy promoting behavioral change runs the risk of having only limited impact.

How is meaning about food formed? Consumer markets play an undeniable role, shaping our food preferences significantly. The interviews I conducted with young folks testify to this fact. Their lives are immersed in this commercial realm. Young people eat a truly staggering number of meals out. Food is largely sorted in terms of commercial brand: Subway is regarded as healthy, Burger King, not healthy. I remember when I first began this project, my daughter, then seven, and I were watching TV and a Subway commercial came on clearly marketed to preteens called "The Power to Choose." The commercial begins with the voiceover of a well-known preteen actress: "Everything's decided for me: when to get up, what to wear, what to read, and of course, when to go to bed." As the commercial runs, we are presented with a series of images of the girl: struggling to get out of bed; her mother's reproach for her punk-inspired outfit; doing math homework in her bedroom. In the commercial's final scene the girl stands at the Subway counter poised to place her order as she proudly declares, "But at Subway I have the power to choose and I eat it up." At the commercial's end, my daughter leapt from the floor declaring, "I want to go to Subway!" The content of the commercial rather than the food itself generated my daughter's enthusiasm. Indeed, marketers from food and beverage industries have been hugely successful in aligning consumption of an infinite number of processed foods—7-UP, Lucky Charms, Cheetos, Capri Sun (Respect the Pouch!), and Hot Pockets, to name but a few—with particular social meanings that resonate with young people: empowerment, freedom, irony, and irreverence.

While the appeal of eating junk food can certainly be explained by the fact that it is rich in salt, sugar, and fat, as well as heavily marketed, it is also a means to solidify young people's identity as being different from adults'—bound up in belonging and membership in age-based groups, which are socially, not biologically, structured. Eating bad food, on the fly, is what you do during final exams. As with an all-nighter, the story is recounted to friends as evidence of student suffering, sacrifice, and dedication to studies. In this sense, eating is performative, and food can be an important staging prop.

For young people, food's cultural logic is both idiosyncratic and patterned, shaped by institutional context and social milieu and informed by a range of identity considerations. Adolescent girls in the Victorian era, as historian Joan Jacobs Brumberg shows us, used food refusal as a means to exercise control and to manage sexual meaning tied to the female body and respectability.[22] For young women who are involved in the pro-ana movement, a contemporary and mostly online community forum in support of an anorexic lifestyle, the denial of food is a moral claim about the strength of resolve and the exercise of restraint—high-premium American cultural values.[23] For a number of the young women I interviewed, who carefully distanced themselves from the adolescent girl who worries obsessively over food and her weight because "that girl" is a poster child for low self-esteem and powerlessness, and is often thought to be too concerned about the evaluations of others, I often heard bold declarations: "I eat." "I like food." "Food is good." One girl, when I asked her what her favorite food was, laughed and replied, "Food is my favorite." While I heard very few young women explicitly talk about dieting, many expressed concern for healthy eating in a way that suggests that health talk is often a foil obscuring what is really a set of concerns with diet and body image for girls.[24] Kristen, who recently swore off Chipotle, explains her rationale: "I feel like for health reasons, just like not health, I'm trying to get in shape. I don't know, just like appearance." "How many calories, how much fat is in that?" as one high school girl explained. "I get grossed out just thinking about it, especially from all those health projects, oh my god! I always think about health." Health discourse, in this sense, is a way for girls to talk about traditional feminine concerns with calories and fat without running the risk of being characterized as the type of girl who is overly concerned with such trifling matters as caring too much about what you look like or what others think. Their words speak to the extent to which our growing preoccupation with health can serve to discipline and constrain the self, perhaps especially for women and girls. I also spoke with many girls who refused to be concerned with health, proudly recalling their unhealthy food habits, and often suspected that they were actually rejecting the conventional feminine concerns about the body. In this way, girls' engagement with food is also an engagement with gender.[25]

At the same time, food is often an afterthought; many young people, in part because of their age, really did not care that much about food and preferred to save their money for more coveted items. As one young woman explained, "I try not to spend money on food if I don't have to. I'd rather spend money on clothes." For many, balancing work, school, and a range of extracurricular activities, eating something other than fast food requires too much of their time, which is often in short supply. In talking about cooking at home, I often heard remarks like, "I don't have time," "I'm pretty cheap," "I hate spending money on groceries." As one college student explained, cooking "takes too long. . . . It's not like I don't enjoy cooking. It's just not convenient." College students especially placed an enormous premium on ease and were more likely to report having a bad diet than high school students in this study. As one college sophomore explained, "I would just get a crap ton of junk food." "Junk food" was often collapsed with "typical college stuff" and thus is conceived of as part and parcel of a particular stage in life. Most young people I spoke to did anticipate an eventual shift where cooking at home would occupy more of their time as they transitioned fully into adulthood—though one does wonder if that expectation will be realized, given the demands of work they are likely to confront as they transition to adulthood.[26]

To be sure, young people's relationships to food are complex. This is the case because a host of social forces shape these relations. Yet, the way youth food consumption is differently structured along regional, ethno-racial, class, and gender lines, the systems of value through which meaning is created, and the way youth food consumption is mediated by larger social practices and processes extending beyond immediate local settings are understudied. This becomes most evident when one compares the dearth of research on *youth* food consumption to an otherwise robust field of food scholarship encompassing studies in the political economy of food and the way food meaning and practice is structured along race-ethnic, national, gender, and class lines in adult society.[27] *Fast-Food Kids* utilizes a range of qualitative research strategies, including participant observation in school cafeterias and fast-food settings, in-depth and focus-group interviews with high school and college-age youth, written narratives about family and food by young people, and analysis of contemporary media and food policy documents, to map the contemporary food landscape as it is lived by young people. I make use of the literatures focused on the political economy of food, the social organization of food consumption, and the social relationship of food to the body and modern subjectivity, all belonging to the emerging field of food and critical nutrition studies, while also drawing upon the conceptual tools of cultural sociology and critical youth studies.[28]

The Moral Weight of Food: Health Food vs. Junk Food

Youth food consumption (of the fast, cheap, and processed variety), whether occurring at home, in school, or at a McDonald's after school, increasingly occupies a morally charged sphere of meaning. Cultural brokers, from parents and advocates for junk-food-free schools to members of food-justice movements, public health researchers and the antihunger lobby, all have much at stake here. From anorexia to obesity, seemingly opposite poles, the youthful body has emerged as a highly contested site upon which cultural categories and moral meanings about national well-being, public and corporate interests, health and risk, and changes to the social organization of everyday life in late modernity are given expression. In market and health policy discourse as well as our everyday talk, youth as a group and childhood as an identity category are symbolized through food choice and consumption.[29] One only has to think for a moment about the classification scheme of "good food" and "bad food," moral categories that align in such a way that kids' food is almost always regarded as "bad" food. The endless iterations of terms like "typical kid fare" and "kid-friendly food" and the constant collapsing of kids' food with junk food has become self-referential—assuming a sort of truth of their own. The trope of the veracious junk-food-consuming teenager (usually male) is a familiar one in popular culture and in debates surrounding the place of food in young people's lives. I admit I was sometimes confounded by the curious food choices of young people (young men especially). I can recall one young man in his first year of community college explaining that the day before he had had six Red Bulls (a high-caffeine energy drink) and a TV dinner for breakfast, followed by half of a banana cream pie his dad had made, having forsaken lunch altogether. Yet, the easy conflation of "kids' food" and "junk food" serves to obscure the range of social forces that shape the contemporary food landscape where young people eat, while also limiting the identity-making possibilities for young people of their food consumption. Young people are often straitjacketed by and tethered to a framework that presumes that biology determines adolescent desires and behavior. Biology is often a prevailing frame in the way we talk about young people and food. So taken for granted, it emerged again and again in interviews, suggesting its influence over the way young people understand their own food practices. As one boy explained, "So, you know, three teenage boys in the house. I mean we'd go through three to four gallons of milk a week. We would just demolish food." I sometimes overheard boys complain about portion size at the school lunch line: "That's it? I'm gonna starve." Though I do not want to minimize the often significant physiological changes and growth in play during adolescence, I do want to caution against a biological criterion as explanatory basis. We need to be careful not to presume that food choice is driven by the all-too-familiar naturalizing refrain "biology is destiny" when thinking through adolescent food consumption. Young people's experiences with food are profoundly social in nature. Rather than thinking about youth consumption as a set of discrete behaviors expressing a biologically rooted developmental trajectory, *Fast-Food Kids* examines youth food consumption as a realm of social meaning, a symbolic sphere through which identities and a complex of social relations materialize, and through which conceptions of childhood are contested, played with, and worked through—by both youth and adults.

Cultural ideas about the meaning of childhood as being distinct from that of adulthood are manifest in the way food is sorted. Take, for example, the fact that much was imputed by the media when President Obama's daughters first enrolled in the elite D.C. private school Sidwell Friends because of the school's lunch menu, which includes items such as fennel and arugula salad with parmesan, curried chicken salad, organic pear and gorgonzola salad, and grilled Portobello mushrooms. How's that for school lunch? New ideas about childhood butt up against old ideas as the status of the child is subject to a historical shift. The playful and mocking tone of media commentary on this story rested on the expectation that sophisticated tastes and food entitlements—that is, what is appropriate for adults and what is appropriate for children to consume—are sorted in terms of a value scale in which class and age are collapsed and used interchangeably. In terms of value schema, food and childhood belong to a sacred realm, each conjuring significant moral sentiment.[30] Yet their sacred value, or "sacralization," to borrow a term from the sociologist Viviana Zelizer, is cast in such a way as to exist in a chronic state of potential collapse as both teeter precariously above possible contamination and defilement by a profane world of corrupting commercial influence. In this sense, youth food consumption is a "morally mediated form of consumption" belonging to "a moral economy."[31]

Nowhere can we see the moral weight of food more clearly than as it has unfolded in recent years around the issue of childhood obesity, an enormously complex issue that reflects an obdurate reality, a measurable phenomenon, and ideological motivations. While childhood obesity is not the focus of this project, *Fast-Food Kids* does seek to complicate our discussions about youth and food and thus inform the way we collectively respond to calls to reduce childhood obesity, as it draws attention to the different levels of social organization that pattern where youth eat, what they eat, and what food has come to mean. *Fast-Food Kids* brackets, in the phenomenological sense, childhood obesity, in order to ward against its reification. Anti-obesity rhetoric, policy, and interventions are an important part of the backdrop of the contemporary food landscape.[32] As a discursive idea, "childhood obesity" circulates widely today, galvanizing action at the individual and institutional level. Different stakeholders, as they mobilize around the *childhood obesity frame* as a public problem, have harnessed its power for their own ends.³³ In the language of semiotics, "childhood obesity" is a floating signifier, such that military leaders have been able to frame childhood obesity in terms of national security risk; and at the same time urban community health activists, a very different group with a different set of priorities, have seized the childhood obesity frame as a means to confront food insecurity in their communities and work against the degradation of public space, including community parks and playgrounds. Educational policy actors were successful in applying pressure to the federal government to increase reimbursement dollars for the National School Lunch Program under the banner of eradicating childhood obesity. And then there are the marketers for children's snack foods who have capitalized on childhood obesity to gain greater market share in the highly competitive processed-food market, with an emphasis on "healthy" and "better for you" as part of recent advertising campaigns.

Childhood obesity as a cultural and historically specific idea is powerful in its diffusion, such that weight has become a major agenda item at yearly wellness visits at many pediatric offices and teachers feel compelled to ban sugary drinks from their classrooms, having identified fruits and whole grains as "appropriate" school snacks and having requested that chips and candy remain at home. As a parent, I can appreciate this as an admirable effort of local schools to positively reshape young people's relationships to food. As a parent, I also admit that I have grown tired of the succession of birthday cupcakes (how many birthdays can you celebrate in one school year?) and the regular round of candy inducements for just about any positive behavior displayed in school. But I have little hope that "fruit kabobs," as one teacher proposed, could actually serve as a reasonable alternative to sprinkles and frosting and the welcomed break from the monotony of the school day such a treat signifies for kids.

We have fixed our individual and collective anxieties on the obese child. We must ask why. What purpose does it serve for us? Think back to my earlier mention of childhood obesity as a national security risk. Congressional testimony has noted that a high and ever-growing percentage of young people are in fact ineligible to serve in the military because they have been designated as too overweight,[34] suggesting then that childhood obesity is tied to the fate of our nation and our ability to remain competitive on a global scale. Whether true or not, this claim certainly signals a set of economic and political priorities and interests in play and a particular orientation to the future. As French sociologist Pierre Bourdieu once remarked, "Health is a disposition toward future."[35]

Many scholars have noted that the rapidly growing concern for childhood obesity has developed in a specific historical period where new strategies of governance demand a self-disciplining citizenry and an ethos of personal responsibility over a collective one, rewarding those who conform and penalizing those who don't or who can't. A number of social scientists have argued persuasively that the panic around childhood obesity is bundled up with new forms of governance centered on the body and body control, what scholars following after Michel Foucault have termed "biopolitics."[36] Incessant talk about health and betterment through lifestyle choice produces a sort of disciplining control whereby the individual aligns her behavior to fit with a prevailing discourse of dietary health, lest she be cast as delinquent in the care of the self.[37] In the words of Kathleen Lebesco, "[T]he language of health and risk has become a repository of a new kind of moralism," with the self as a site of "ongoing moral transformation."[38] In this context, a disciplined, self-reliant, and enterprising citizen who is in command of her own trajectory is valorized. She is neither beholden to nor reliant on collective entities such as government, nor is she enslaved to her own desire, and in this sense, she is free.

Critical nutritional scholar Charlotte Biltekoff demonstrates that campaigns aimed at "improving people's eating habits" have long been seen by social reformers "as a way to improve their moral character."[39] In this sense the current focus on childhood obesity reflects "the social valence of eating right over the last century," at the same time expressing a new set of social considerations that have found expression in our focus on dietary health.[40] A number of cultural critics and scholars have rightly identified a narrowing of our gaze on obesity as symptomatic of broader political, economic, and cultural currents that coalesce around a changing set of social relationships of state and the individual. This shift is often associated with a neoliberal project that privileges personal responsibility, a declining investment in any notion of the "public" as binding, and a trend toward privatization of what were once regarded as public goods, including school lunch programs.[41] In what is often called a neoliberal era, empowerment is thought to largely reside in individuals and not collectives; *personal* empowerment is thought to be the most effective pathway to social change.

The obese body is cast as anathema to a neoliberal imperative that demands a citizenry that is self-regulating and disciplined, what Biltekoff calls "the unhealthy other."[42] In this context, the fit body is idealized, and moral judgments about deviant bodies intensify. It is also in this context that prescriptions for self-change proliferate. "Health," itself, "is a term replete with value judgments, hierarchies and blind assumptions that speak as much about power and privilege as they do about well-being," argues sociologists Jonathan Metzel and Anna Kirkland.[43] Obese children are often cast as victims of their own deficits—seen to lack self-control, with parents demonized as too incompetent, too uncaring, or too indulgent to teach their children "to make good choices." Recall the child who in 2011 was removed from the care of his mother by the state courts on the grounds of medical neglect because he was too large.[44] In this case, responsibility for obesity rests entirely with the mother and the choices she makes, independent of a social context. In addition to gender stereotypes, racial and class stereotypes are often invoked, as well as a deep-rooted racial and class bias that presumes that white, middle-class parents are morally superior ones.[45]

Campaigns to reverse obesity trends among the young sometimes look more like a crusade against fat, giving rise to what anthropologist Susan Greenhalgh has termed "bio-bullying," wherein overweight kids whose bodies do not conform to that of the fit, self-disciplined citizen-in-the-making are the subject of increasing scrutiny and "a new freedom among the general public to demonize fatness under the aegis of 'health' is commonplace."[46] Few antibullying school initiatives include as part of their programming a focus on fat, but perhaps they should.

As a cultural idea, childhood obesity is impossible to separate from our moral and aesthetic judgments. The overt moralizing tone in talk about childhood obesity, itself a mechanism of social control, is widespread, while the ability to recognize it as such is often lost on us. As childhood obesity has gained greater traction, it has become increasingly difficult to parse out a public health concern with childhood obesity from a moral rhetoric focused on long-standing American values of self-care and self-reliance and our cultural disdain for lifestyles that depart from middle-class ways of being.

Yet as much as childhood obesity is bound to a moral sphere of meaning, childhood obesity in the world of public health is presumed to exist in objectified form, as a set of discrete numbers. Supported by the weight of an ever-churning stream of statistics, it is taken as fact, with little reflection given to the motivation or warrant for intervention that obesity statistics, as numerical claims, serve to bolster.[47] While I am happy to leave the work of enumeration to other social scientists and public health researchers, let me again stress caution in our quick rush to lay blame on the numerous woes of weight. It behooves us to proceed cautiously as we respond to what can be alarmist rhetoric around childhood obesity as epidemic. As food scholar Julie Guthman wisely proclaims, obesity requires social explanation and medical explanation.

Critical nutrition studies, with its focus on "nutrition as a cultural practice that both shapes and is shaped by other cultural practices taking into account issues of power, identity and ideology,"[48] has been particularly attentive to understanding the moral weight of food and how it can be used to govern. Critical nutrition and health scholars also recognize that disparities in health and well-being are a part of the obesity puzzle. It is worth noting here that the majority of children and adolescents who are classified as obese are not low income; however, obesity prevalence decreases as income and education increase: poor children have a higher obesity risk than higher-income children, which suggests that inequality is an important part of understanding the causes of obesity.[49] There are very real and deepening health disparities arising from place-based inequalities, which are also related to racial segregation, that have been well documented.[50] Take, for example, poor urban areas where fear of crime drives many indoors in front of the TV and out of public parks, and where access to nutritious food requires a level of ingenuity often beyond human possibility since there are so few grocery stores nearby[51]—or rural poor communities where travel to grocery stores to purchase fresh fruits and vegetables presumes access to a car, or money for gas. In such ways, health and risk are spatially structured, tied to issues of immobility, segregation and isolation, and lack of resources and opportunities.[52] As nutrition scholar Marion Nestle has observed, "[P]overty continues to be the single most important danger signal for nutritional deficiencies in American children."[53] For young people, health disparities, usually manifestations of income disparities, spatial location, a legacy of racial segregation, or some combination of the three, have been linked to a number of negative outcomes, including school readiness, academic performance, and greater likelihood of dropping out of high school.[54] It is the case that some communities, usually those that are poor, isolated, and of color, run a higher risk of diet-related health problems than others, and this has little to do with moral values but instead results from economic and social policy, social support and social networks, access to transportation, and the economic opportunity determined by where youth live.[55]

Where Kids Eat

Fast-Food Kids explores what food reveals about the cultural and economic factors of young people's lives as they move from home to school to commercial settings. Yale's Rudd Center on Food Policy and Obesity's *Fast-Food Facts: Evaluating Fast-Food Nutrition and Marketing* reports that one-third of children in the United States get 17 percent of their caloric intake from fast food every day.[56] "Eighty-four percent of parents reported taking their child to a fast-food restaurant at least once in the past week; and 66% reported going to McDonald's."[57] In 2013, 40 percent of teenagers consumed fast food every day.[58] The fact that so much time is spent eating fast foods is hardly surprising given that in 2010 an estimated $4.2 billion was spent by fast-food industries on advertising.[59] Children and adolescents represent a key target market, with African American and Hispanic children disproportionately targeted, according to the Rudd Center. The way food is marketed exercises a significant influence over the foods youth choose. But it is not simply a matter of young people and their parents seeking out commercial foods; commercial foods worm their way into the very places where most of young people's lives unfold—that is, home and school, institutional arenas thought to exist outside the world of commercial influence and market forces.[60]

Public schools have failed to avoid the influence of marketization and commercial creep as public resources for education recede and transnational food corporations and their political counterpart, the GMA (the Grocer's Manufacturers Association, a powerful food and beverage lobby), provide funding to schools, stocking their lunchroom freezers and school vending machines. These machines, which dispense, at a minimum cost, low-nutritional-value food and drinks, are mainstays of American high school cafeterias; only in 2013 were federal nutritional guidelines established for them. Schools face a double bind because in the absence of resources, they depend on vending machines as a lucrative revenue stream. In 2003 in Texas alone, vending machines produced $54 million in revenue for schools, and companies cashed in on this easy sell.[61] Soft drink companies have long brokered exclusive and often unequal contracts that enable "pouring rights" with school districts, obligating schools to sell their sodas in vending machines and at school events in exchange for the dangling carrot of "free" educational resources.[62] Since most public schools have no allotted food budgets apart from reimbursements from the National School Lunch Program, food directors are reliant on sales of what are called competitive foods (e.g., Otis Spunkmeyer cookies, Rice Krispy treats, Pop-Tarts, Doritos) to break even.[63] In the wake of a declining public investment in schools, many food companies have realized the sizeable market share to be gained and have aggressively partnered with schools. Consider Krispy Kreme's "Doughnuts for A's" program, whereby every A awarded earns the student a free doughnut. Advertising for Lay's potato chips, Oreo cookies, and Rockstar energy drinks can be found on book covers and educational posters in high schools across America, as can "healthy" foods, such as Dole pineapple. Advertising in schools is ubiquitous, but is largely taken for granted. Many advocates for school food reform have worked diligently to highlight the connection between nutritious, healthy eating and academic performance, exposing the glaring irony of a public educational mission at odds with a public health mission.[64]

Readily recognizable commercial fast foods and processed snack items are woven into the everyday fabric of school. Perhaps one of the most straightforward instances of branded fast foods' presence in school I came across was at a private high school I visited a few times during lunch over the course of my research for this project. The school,

Piedmont, which caters mostly to upper-income families, is without a working kitchen. Absent a kitchen or kitchen staff, the PTA, comprised almost entirely of mothers, has partnered with local fast-food franchises Chick-fil-A, Honey Baked Ham, and Domino's pizza to provide student lunches several days a week. The franchises make the food, the PTA moms serve it, and parents pay for it. Students submit menu selections in advance of the lunch with their payment, which can runs upwards of eight dollars per meal, with the exception of Domino's pizza, which is much cheaper. The mothers volunteer their time (though they refuse to wear the standard hairnets kitchen workers are required to wear), handing out lunches during the lunch period, and the small margin they gain is used to cover the PTA's operating budget.

How we got overly processed, energy-dense, nutritionally poor commercial foods in school is a long and complicated story. Sociologist Janet Poppendieck's *Free for All: Fixing School Food in America,* which examines the rapid rise of competitive foods (also called à la carte items) in the last quarter of the twentieth century, shows how the food and beverage industries were able to exploit a weakening system of government funding and regulation for school lunch, transforming what passed as food in school cafeterias.[65] These revenue-driven foods—nachos, Doritos, Rice Krispies Treats, Pop-Tarts—because they are excluded from the federal reimbursable meal program, operated until very recently beyond the reach of federal oversight.[66] Much of this has passed unnoticed as kids moved through lunch lines. Kids may complain about the food, but apart from these intermittent grumblings, it is all a matter of course. As Dan, the food director from one of the public schools I observed for this project, opined, "Everybody always forgets the food."

Transformations in the National School Lunch Program (NSLP) in the late 1970s set the conditions for an influx of market-driven, overly processed foods, what Poppendieck has called "carnival fare." While the NSLP, established in 1946, was originally a program conceived to feed all of our nation's children nutritious meals to promote a healthy citizenry, in the 1970s it converted to a program of poor food for poor kids. In an effort to reduce government spending during the '70s and '80s, federal dollars for school lunch waned and so did student participation, especially among middle-class children, since the federal government was suddenly much less willing to subsidize their lunch. A larger number of middle-class students withdrew from a program that was increasingly defined as a program for the poor, with the heavy weight of stigma attached. This resulted in a significant loss in revenue. With declining revenues, school lunch programs were forced to economize, to cut corners on taste and nutrition to overcome budget shortfalls. Enter competitive foods.[67] These foods are not included in the NSLP but are an important source of revenue for lunchrooms; their ubiquity in school lunchrooms reflects public schools' heavy reliance on the commercial food industry's offerings of cheap, processed, and nutritionally poor foods to meet their operating costs.[68] Healthy and nutritious meals, as part of a public food-provisioning system, became even more difficult to come by.[69] As Poppendieck writes,

> Our spectacular failure to provide fresh, appealing, healthy meals for all our children is the result of a series of specific and identifiable social choices that we have made: a massive disinvestment in our public schools, an industrialized food system, an agriculture policy centered on subsidies for large-scale commodity production, a business model rather than a public health approach to school food programs.[70]

While reforms in the public school food system to address the presence and influence of commercial entities are underway with efforts to tighten nutritional standards, for example, these efforts have also been met with a significant counteroffensive by different commercial players. Public records reveal that food and beverage industries spent $175 million between 2009 and 2011 alone to lobby against tougher nutritional standards for food marketed to children, to ensure that exercise drinks could still be found in high school vending machines, even if soda can't, and to guarantee that french fries remain on the menu in public schools as part of the National School Lunch Program.[71] Consider also the hefty financial muscle exercised by what is sometimes called "big soda" to defeat the proposed excise tax on soda in Washington, D.C., a tax that was intended to defray costs associated with the 2010 D.C. Healthy Schools Act.[72] This larger complex of arrangements serves as a backdrop for understanding youth's food consumption in school, and thus warrants serious investigation.

Public schools are not the only institutional setting increasingly shaped by commercial forces. Family arrangements also have been subject to increasing marketization, radically reconfiguring the family meal, for example. The accelerating pace of life for a large number of Americans has meant transformation in both food production and food consumption. Shared meal times have declined over the last several decades as families confront a range of transformations that impinge on the quotidian dimensions of family life, with snacking emerging in its place. Janet Poppendieck notes that "speed and preparation ease" are primary consideration in meal planning today.[73] The 2009 American Community Survey of the U.S. Census reveals that less than 60 percent of parents surveyed reported having dinner with their twelve- to seventeen-year-old children daily during a typical week.[74] Young people's increased obligations outside the home, especially among upper-income youth, combined with parental work demands, impose upon shared meal times, with consequences for the way family members understand the nature of collective life at home. As sociologist Arlie Hochschild has argued, "[J]ust as market conditions ripened the soil for capitalism, so a weakened family prepares the soil for a commercialized spirit of domestic life."[75]

These changes in family life are compounded by the changing economic realities of so many families who labor to put food, any food, on their family table. Millions of Americans continued in 2012 to struggle to afford enough food, according to food hardship data from the Food Research and Action Center (FRAC).[76] To be more precise, one in six Americans (18 percent) said in 2012 that there had been times over the preceding twelve months when they did not have enough money to buy food that they or their families needed. This is well illustrated in the powerful 2012 documentary *A Place at the Table*, which chronicles the struggles of "the new hungry," or those considered to be "food insecure." While older forms of hunger were a result of food shortages, captured in the haunting images of Depression-era breadlines, the new hunger is not marked by an absence of food necessarily but by an absence of nutrient-rich foods.[77] In the wake of declines in government food assistance and the rise of charity-based food donations, those who are food insecure and rely on charitable food giving rarely suffer from shortages of crackers, cookies, chips, packaged ramen noodles, peanut butter, and other food items that have a long shelf-life, since they represent the bulk of donated foods.[78]

While for families with resources, their busy lives drive them into the commercial worlds of the drive-through, processed snacks, and ready-made meals, for families at the other economic end, a different set of circumstance is in play. Thus, whereas the accelerating pace of daily life helps to explain how the middle and upper-middle classes eat, for the poor, especially for the young and old, boredom, immobility, and deacceleration often characterize their daily routines. Middle- and upper-income kids in the suburbs, where much of this research was completed, busily move from activity to activity, grabbing something that approximates a meal in between. But this is not the case for poor kids, whose afternoons instead are often spent passing the time at McDonald's, bored and often stranded, waiting for the last school bus to take them home.

Yet, despite changes in the economic realities and time burdens of American families, food preparation and consumption remain expressions of intimacy and care, even as both activities have been radically altered by large-scale economic processes, among them changing work-family patterns, the movement of large numbers of women into the work force, the geographical dispersal of family units, the expansion of commercial markets, and the outsourcing to those markets of responsibilities historically performed at home.

The complicated relationships among markets, material constraints, and meaning are what I seek to better understand in *Fast-Food Kids*. School food, uniformly characterized as bad, for instance, reflects our deep cultural ambivalence about the public provisioning of food to children. We largely associate feeding children with the private sphere of home, motherly care, and the durable bonds of family. And while school food assumes a sort of mythic status as "gross," home-cooked food is locked in what historian Stephanie Coontz terms "the nostalgia trap."[79] As both a private *and* a public good, food is entangled with a moral sphere of sentimentality and care and also an economic sphere of production, exchange, and consumption. Of course, these two spheres of activity, as sociologist Viviana Zelizer has repeatedly shown, are not so neatly divided in the actual world as they are in our thinking.[80] In the actual realm of daily interaction and institutional practice, economic transactions and sentiment are falsely separated. Instead, the arrangements within these spheres of social meaning are convoluted, complicated, and contradictory. In the case of food, this is especially glaring.

Food is a moral object, an economic object, an object of play, and an aesthetic object, bound to multiple registers of health and well-being. As food travels across private (home) and public spheres of social life (community, school, consumer realm), family, and peer group, its meaning and value transform. The exchange of french fries in the commercial realm, for example, often has more to do with status displays and tests of friendship for youth than with market logics (recall the girls sharing the single sundae at Baskin-Robbins recounted at the chapter's beginning). Markets and the social meanings that flow from them play an ever-expanding role in the lives of youth at home, at school, and in the spaces in between, often sites we regard as noncommercial, even if in truth they are not and never have been.

Yet as we talk about food in an institutional setting, we are more likely to look to macro-level processes to understand them. And as important as it is to understand how industrial agriculture and government food policy has transformed what kids eat in school, such a focus often overlooks the meaning-making activities that both inspire and constrain action in these institutional realms. Thus, while a core aim of this project is to map how moral categories and commercial logics have come to shape youth's food consumption at home and at school, *Fast-Food Kids* examines these processes as they are given expression in the local organization of young people's lives as they move through lunch lines in their school cafeteria, order a #2 at McDonald's, or eat their reheated dinner alone, in front of the television, as they complete the last leg of homework after returning home from basketball practice long after other family members have eaten. The way these changes are understood and experienced by young people themselves is important to understand as they organize their activities in and beyond home, in and around school, and has relevance for the way we address concerns about young people's food consumption and health as scholars and advocates for food policy change.

The Study

The idea for this project emerged in late 2007 while I was involved with another interview-based project on youth that didn't seem to be going anywhere. I entered the field in 2008 with only a small inkling of where this project might lead me and the questions I might answer. As with my other ethnographic projects, which also focused on youth, the first on high school proms and the second on youth and cars, I was interested in taking a single object or event that on the surface appears trivial but upon closer inspection of the meanings, social relationships, and cultural logics around it reveals deep cultural significance. High school proms, cars, and fast food all provide opportunities to explore mediations on consumer culture, how it refracts in cultural scenes and settings out of which everyday life is built. So I began with an open mind, a pen and pad, and a few projects behind me, and went to a McDonald's only to discover a robust social space. I returned to that McDonald's for several years, while also expanding my observational field to include a number of other fast-food settings where kids gather en masse directly following the end of the school day. Settings were selected on the basis of proximity to public high schools. In total, two Subways, one Baskin-Robbins, one Dairy Queen, four McDonald's restaurants, two Chipotles, three Starbucks stores, and one Baja Fresh were observed, with sustained observations conducted at four McDonald's settings and one Chipotle from 2008 to 2010.

Pretty early on in the project I decided I wanted to look at food and the relationships formed around food across different institutional fields—school, family, the commercial realm—to map in the tradition of multisited ethnography the connections between and across fields. In this sense, I have been less concerned with comparative dimensions of the project (how kids eat at home, how kids eat in a commercial setting, how kids eat at school) and more interested in understanding how the logics and practices that constitute these institutional settings, which themselves are not truly separate, bleed into one another, shaping and organizing the practices of each. The pull of the commercial food realm, for example, is as much about the push of packed family schedules and bad school food as it is about the food itself or its marketing. In this sense, the private provisioning of foods historically undertaken in the home and our increasing inability to do that work, combined with our deep cultural ambivalence toward food as a public good, help to push young folks toward the commercial realm and its food offerings. To understand youth consumption of commercial foods, then, we must also understand the meaning of food as it is consumed in other spheres of social life. And thus, systematic observations in school and commercial settings came to represent a core part of this project. I spent several month observing school lunches at two public high schools: Thurgood High School in the fall of 2010 and Washington High School in the spring of 2010. In different ways, as I undertook my observations, each school was at the forefront of school food reforms inspired by a call for improved dietary health. Thurgood and Washington belong to different school districts, but both are public. They provide interesting points of comparison owing to differences in the cultural and economic base of students, the schools' academic records, and each food director's vision and commitments. Thurgood High School enrolls twenty-two hundred tenth-, eleventh-, and twelfth-grade students and is ethnically and racially diverse, with 43 percent of the students being African American, 27 percent Hispanic, 21 percent white, and 7 percent Asian/Pacific Islander and American Indian.[81] Washington High School enrolls just over eight hundred eighth- through twelfth-grade students and is less diverse racially and economically, with 73 percent of its students being white, 6 percent African American, 9 percent Hispanic, and 11 percent Asian/Pacific Islander. Washington has been nationally ranked for the last decade as a top public school, while in 2010 Thurgood was awarded by the U.S. Department of Education the unlucky designation "persistently low-achieving school." Both schools are located in relatively wealthy communities in a major metropolitan area, but in the case of Thurgood, a large base of students is bused in from the district's periphery, where lower-income and subsidized housing is concentrated. At Thurgood in 2010, around 60 percent of students were on free or subsidized lunch, while less than 8 percent of students at Washington were. Both schools' cafeterias are settings where larger narratives about market influence in school settings, cultural discourses on health, and gender, class, and racial inequalities come to bear, structuring the types of interactions that unfold therein. A third school (private) was visited, though only a few times, as a point of interest because they had no working kitchen and relied heavily on the PTA to organize lunch.[82]

Fast-Food Kids also draws on interviews and focus groups conducted with fifty-six young adults (aged fifteen to twenty-three) representing different economic situations, family forms, and racial/ethnic groups, as well as a small collection of adults involved in community- based food work. Principles of theoretical sampling guided interview procedures. Interview and focus-group participants were recruited through purposive and convenience sampling, with the explicit purpose of developing a racially and economically diverse pool of respondents; I included youth enrolled in high school, community college, and four-year college because I was particularly interested to understand how school figures in youth's food lives. Like the observations, all interviews were conducted with young people residing in a major metropolitan area, with recruitment occurring in some cases from the observational sites. What this means is that the experiences of rural youth are not represented in these pages, but instead youth living in and around a city and its surrounding suburbs. I consider this a meaningful omission and hope other scholars will work to fill that lacuna. Focus-group and in-depth interviews with young adults allowed me to gain a sense of the cultural significance youth attach to food consumption in school, at home, and in commercial settings from the perspective of young people themselves, a group whose perspectives rarely inform policy discussions or interventions.

Another rich data source upon which this analysis rests is written narratives collected about family life and food beginning in 2007. I amassed just over 260 one-page narratives about family food memories written by college students between the ages of eighteen and twenty-three. The written narratives offer a window into the practical and symbolic dimensions of contemporary family life as understood and narrated by young people, revealing what young people, on the cusp of adulthood, think about families of the present, their own and others, as they make sense of the internal transformations in families as children grow older, families migrate and move, parents divorce and remarry, and mothers return to work. These narratives served as a meaningful supplement to interview data and are the primary basis of the analysis in chapter 1, focusing on food provisioning at home.

A broad range of policy and media materials focused on local and national food reforms that impact young people were also collected. Close analysis of contemporary documents relating to youth, food, and public health initiatives has allowed me to trace the language and framing of policy and public discourse with its current focus on childhood obesity and its impact on the work of school food directors in schools.

While the focus of this research is youth, *Fast-Food Kids* also investigates the institutional conditions in which kids articulate their relationship to food.

The Book

Each of the chapters zeroes in on a particular aspect of youth and the changing food landscape— school, home, and commercial realm—with attention to three core tensions through which youth food consumption as a sphere of social meaning is created and ultimately understood. The first core tension takes shape around two competing frames: the first casts food as a private good, rooted deeply in relations of home tied to our most durable social bonds, and the second casts food as a public good, and thus part of a public provisioning system of care to which we are collectively obligated. A second and related tension takes shape around food as gift, and thus part of the symbolic order, and food as commodity, arising from an economic order. This tension points to how food is an objectified form shaped by economic and relational imperatives. The final tension exists between food as an object of play, central to youth cultural worlds, identity making in school, and the commercial realm, and food as an object of care through which intimate ties of home and social ties in and to the public institution of school are forged. These three tensions—gift/commodity, public good/private good, and play/care—are explored across the chapters.

Chapter 1 explores food and family life, focusing on changes to modern families as expressed in the interviews and narratives about family meals as a form of private food provisioning that is increasingly shaped by tensions between commodified social relations on the one hand and food as object of care, tied to a gift exchange between parents and children, on the other. This chapter documents the symbolic currency of longing and belonging for young people as they talk about food and family life, with the aim to examine the tension between family as a sphere of practical activity and family as symbolic sphere, both shaped by processes of marketization that prevail in the period of late capitalism. The next three chapters follow young people as they travel from home to school, and thus examine food as it is transformed from a private good to a public good.

Chapter 2 examines what is on the lunch menu at Thurgood High School, focusing on the work of Brenda, Thurgood's food director, and her effort to bring into being a public food-provisioning system promoting students' recognition and respect alongside dietary health. Chapter 3 returns to Thurgood's lunchroom, exploring food as an object through which youth forge relationships to the institution of school and each other. Attention is given to the complex spatial arrangements in the cafeteria and the role food plays in group boundary and social identity making for youth, thereby complicating Brenda's vision of school food as a means to address inequality rather than reproduce it. Chapter 4 focuses on Washington High School and its cafeteria, examining the different types of food found there—commercial food, school food, and food brought from home—and the role parents play in shaping the cafeteria and students, with specific attention to social class and its consequence for a public food provisioning system. All three chapters are organized with an eye to understanding how social inequalities pattern students' relationship to the cafeteria and the food therein, highlighting how social meaning expresses and informs that relationship.

Chapter 5 explores youth food consumption in commercial food settings as youth leave school at the end of the day, focusing in particular on McDonald's and Chipotle as popular after-school destinations. Attention is given to two core elements of youth food consumption in the commercial realm—play and gift exchange—examining the extent to which youth food consumption fulfills youth cultural ends alongside and against commercial market ends. The conclusion to *Fast-Food Kids* considers how we might think about youth food consumption, as a sphere of social meaning constituted in the everyday spaces of school, home, and commercial realms, and its relationship to our democratic future. A discussion of the methodological issues at stake in doing multisited ethnography can be found in the methods appendix.

For an ethnographer, food is one way into the worlds of young people. Studying youth's food consumption as shaped by systems of meaning that hold value in youth cultural worlds promises to shed light on how young people negotiate a set of shifting arrangements in the social organization of school and home, the relations of constraint therein, and the connection between social inequalities in daily life and health and well-being. The meanings young people attach to food as cultural object tell us much about their social world and their place in it.[83] This book is my attempt to demonstrate the value of cultural analysis for a topic that has generated tremendous policy and public interest and to make a case for what greater attention to culture, with its focus on collective meaning, schemes of value, symbolic action, and social interaction, yields for health policy and public decision making.

1

The Family Meal

Eating Together, Eating Apart

The 2009 Hollywood blockbuster *The Blind Side* is an uplifting and sentimental story about Baltimore Ravens defensive tackle Michael Oher and his journey to the NFL as a black, poor teenage boy left homeless by his drug-addicted mother and the woman who helps him get there, Leigh Anne Tuohy, a no-nonsense, wealthy, white southern Christian woman. The movie focuses on unlikely connections, the redemptive power of family love, and the straitjacketed despair of being young, poor, and alone. Theirs is a chance meeting. On a football scholarship Michael attends the private school Tuohy's son and daughter also attend. One evening in the dead of winter Leigh Anne is driving home when she spots Michael walking on the side of a country road in short sleeves and shorts, carrying his only belongings—a balled-up change of clothes in a small plastic grocery bag. Michael is invited to sleep on the Tuohy's couch and the next day is asked to stay for Thanksgiving dinner.

As the Thanksgiving scene begins, we see the two Tuohy children and their father stretched across oversized, comfy couches, eyes fixed to the televised holiday football game, with mother standing at the kitchen counter, a glass of red wine balanced in her hand. "Come-an-get-it, y'all," she calls as she barely lifts her eyes from the magazine she's reading. The two kids and father hop up in anticipation. They serve themselves from the buffet-style arrangement of food on the kitchen counter, eyes racing between the action on the TV and the food itself as steaming heaps of mashed potatoes, collard greens, turkey, and other holiday fixings are piled atop their plates. With a perfunctory nod, the father encourages, "Everyone thank your mother for driving to the store and getting this," and in the sweet southern tones of children raised below the Mason Dixon line, the two reply, "Thank ya Mama," as they fix their gaze back to the screen.

Except, of course, orphaned Michael, who finds a place at the empty table in the formal dining room and quietly eats with his head bowed. This scene of a fractured family sharing the same physical place, together but alone, as each is engaged in solitary activity, depicts an entirely modern moment in the life of American families. The scene hints at a collapse of family as defined by the shared, ceremonial act of eating, and their quiet despair despite the absence of want for material things. Food is abundant but outsourced and thus stripped of its significance as marker of home-grown love. All are engaged in what sociologist Arlie Hochschild has called "collective loafing": the primary relationship of each is to the TV and not each other.[1] Except, of course, Michael, who gestures to the ritual food event we recognize as Thanksgiving as he sits waiting. His act is suggestive of the high symbolic resonance of the so-called traditional family meal.[2] Food has long been a repository of meaning and memory for us as individuals and the collectives to which we belong, most important among them—the durable bonds of family.[3]

To suggest that families are knit together, intimately joined, through food preparation and food consumption is to state the obvious.[4] Family members gather together daily to prepare and consume food. In modern America, this takes a variety of forms as different actors and circumstances impinge upon the act itself.[5] Food provisioning and preparing, the work involved in what sociologist Marj DeVault regards as "feeding the family," has long been recognized as belonging within the matrix of familial care.[6] Yet, many family scholars have noted that the delivery of that care has grown increasingly more complicated and burdened. Arlie Hochschild, for instance, has identified a "growing care gap" whereby "informal systems of kin care have grown more fragile, uncertain, and fragmented" at a time when family life has grown more demanding as we care for young and old in new ways, manage ever-changing relationships arising from blended families, and maintain ties often across vast expanses.[7]

Preparing food and eating have been transformed over the last several decades by shifts in large-scale economic processes and cultural changes, among them changing work-family patterns and the geographical dispersal of family units. The expansion of commercial markets and the outsourcing of responsibilities historically performed within the domestic realm to those markets,[8] the rise of industrial agriculture, and a flooding of ready-to-eat processed foods into the market have all played a significant role in modern family food provisioning.[9]

The movement of large numbers of women into the labor force over the last four decades also helps to explain changes to the food landscape of families.[10] An overall increase in the total number of hours worked among dual-wage-earning families and single parents with children has combined with changing demands and increased obligation for children themselves as they move through childhood in preparation for the adult roles they will later assume.[11] American middle-class children spend an increasing number of weekly hours in structured activities, contributing to the "growing time crunch in families—parents' efforts to schedule children, while they themselves are scheduled."[12]

What is more, the composition of families has changed. In the last several decades we have witnessed a proliferation of different household form—including single-parent, same-sex, extended, and blended families—emerging in place of the married, heterosexual, nuclear family household. It is nearly impossible to talk about a single family form as a norm.[13] The widespread practice of breakups and recoupling, described by sociologist Andrew Cherlin as "the marriage-go-round," offers but one example of the changing rhythms of family life as we move into the twenty-first century.[14] Sociologist Allison Pugh identifies a fundamental shift in the way we understand our most durable social bonds of family, noting an increase in the diversity of relationship forms, alongside a decrease in their duration. In other words, relationships, as varied as they are, just don't last as long as they once did, and this, Pugh argues, reflects a substantial change in the nature of commitment toward what she calls a postindustrial model of "flexible" commitment and a cooling of intimate ties.[15] This shift, she argues, has emerged in response to the increasingly complex demands on the self and the fracturing of our time during the period often termed "late modernity."[16]

The result of these changes is an accelerating pace for daily life for an increasing number of parents *and* their children, which in turn has meant transformation in both food production and food consumption. Shared meal times have waned, and food has declined in *practical* importance for families. As Steve, a twenty-two-year-old full-time student with a full-time job and a two-year-old son, remarked, "I do food on the cheap." Steve described meals bought from 7-Eleven, largely eaten on the fly. These days, "speed and preparation ease are overwhelmingly rated as top considerations in food selection processes," and snacking and meal time are increasingly indistinguishable.[17] Child Trends' policy research databank reports that "as children grow older and become more independent during adolescence, they tend to spend less time with the family and eat more meals away from the home."[18]

Parents' income and education predict the likelihood of parents eating with their children, though in a way that will probably surprise most readers. Today, children in lower-income families, and those whose parents have completed less education, are *more* likely to have meals together with their families than are children with wealthier or more educated parents, according to the American Community Survey, collected by the U.S. Census.[19] Poor families are most likely to eat together, according to the U.S Census.[20] Adolescents with foreign-born parents are also more likely to eat dinner together than those with parents who are not foreign born, though according to the U.S. Census, the family structure, whether single-parent or dual-parent, does not influence the likelihood of eating together.[21]

Yet, as much as food has declined in *practical* importance, it has been elevated in *symbolic* importance.[22] Food prepared in the home is at once an object around which family life materializes in concrete form and an object that operates on a symbolic register as highly sentimentalized. For American families, food preparation and consumption are expressions of intimacy and care. Consider, for example, the now-ubiquitous term "comfort food," invoked in everyday talk and the larger discursive landscape where food is sorted in terms of the emotional return it provides. Comfort food is all about home, care, and a feeling of emotional safety and security—all presumed to be increasingly threatened by large-scale social changes—and, thus, is a social object tied to our collective anxiety. In our collective imagination, home-cooked food is idealized as symbol of the strong, loving family, often obscuring the very real practical constraints of food production at home.

What follows is a look at the place of food in families as it is understood by youth, a group generally thought of as the recipients, rather than the providers, of care.[23] While I found that youth play active roles in food decisions in the home and in some cases food provisioning, they also hold specific expectations for care; that is, adult family members, especially mothers, are supposed to take the lead in providing food for the family as a whole. Young people expressed longing and disappointment when that expectation was not met. This creates a dilemma for parents since providing care through home-cooked meals is increasingly out of reach.

Between 2007 and 2012 I collected just over 260 written narratives about family and food by young adults between the ages of eighteen and twenty-three.[24] This chapter draws largely on those writings, as well as on interviews conducted with young adults. My aim here is to identify how young adults think about food consumption at home, and the systems of value and meaning about care and belonging that inform their perspectives. Their words reveal a marked tension between the precariousness of family life, arising in large part from the economic imperatives of work, and the symbolic work of family members, old and young, to maintain family bonds through family food rituals. Their words encourage us to think more critically about food policy programs that rely too heavily on private systems of food provisioning and care—that is, the food provided and eaten in the private setting of home—calling upon us to think more seriously about care as not simply a private good belonging to family groups but also a public good, delivered within public institutions, such as schools.[25]

The Family Meal

Most memories young people hold about family and food depict moments of family togetherness, care, and love. One writer even titled his family memory "Best Food Experience," even though the only prompt given by me was to write about a single family food memory. The shared family meal for the young people in this study is a central site for the "symbolic, ritualized performances of family values."[26] While some narratives were matter-of-fact and without sentiment—"I grew up on fast-food";[27] "My family ate out often because no one really liked to cook. We would get Pizza Hut pizza every weekend and sometimes we would have McDonald's breakfast on other weekends"[28]—many more were awash with a nostalgia for the rituals of togetherness. Consider these snapshots: "Food reminds me of home";[29] "When we eat and drink together, I feel like I have a wonderful life";[30] "My family felt complete";[31] "Waiting each and every year for that homemade goodness is well deserved when you get to have that first forkful of pie."[32] Referencing Korean Thanksgiving, one writer offered, "made me feel safe, warm, and nourished."[33] "Our mornings were very Beaver Cleaver," one writer explained. "This is so memorable to me because this happened every single morning for several years of my life, it was one of the only times we were all together."[34]

Specific foods were often invested with meaning about family unity and love. "Whenever I think of family, food comes to mind. Sweet potatoes bring my family together."[35] "Our special family dinners centered around our Sunday *asados* . . . . I love the feeling of good Argentinean barbeque because it evokes feelings of family and identity with my Spanish heritage."[36] For these youth, food belongs to the realm of feeling. *Pierogis* (Polish dumplings), *salteñas*, *gajar ka halwa* (sweetened carrot dessert), *pukacapas*, *cuñapés* (Bolivian), borscht, *kabuli*, *wot*, *injera* (Ethiopian), bean paste soup (Korean), ceviche, tamales, moussaka (Egyptian), and fried tilapia (Philippines) acquired special significance because they were seen as an expression of distinct family identities *and* ethnic attachments. Consider the following narrative about Shin Ramyun, a spicy Korean dish, and the meaning it held in terms of family ties amidst disruption and change.

> From preschool to first grade, I lived in an apartment within a poor area. It was next to a busy street and only a few minutes from the highway. By the time I was in second grade we moved into a small single home in a quiet suburb. . . . I remember the first meal I ever had in this house and it was when we first moved in and there was nothing in the house except a refrigerator. . . . There wasn't anything in the refrigerator for us to eat so my mom resorted to making ramen noodles. I was unfortunately very accustomed to eating ramen noodles but this time was different. My mom had only a large pot that we all shared and we ate while sitting on the floor of the kitchen. Eating ramen brings back many memories of eating together with my family.[37]

In some cases, special family food assumed an almost magical quality, its properties able to resolve all manner of trouble. Consider this tale about seaweed soup, a staple of a South Korean diet, made for the first time for this writer, now nineteen, in the first grade, by her mother:

> When I had to take the SATs in high school, I had been struggling with balancing SAT studying, homework, and extra-curricular activities. Therefore when it became time for me to test, I got very nervous. . . . Amazingly, though, right when I saw the seaweed soup, I felt much better. As the soup went down my throat and into my stomach, I could feel the soothing plunge of warmness throughout my body and it began to calm me down. . . . A few weeks later I checked my SAT scores to see how I had done and I had scored the best that I had ever done before![38]

At the end of her narrative she concludes, "Every time my mother makes this seaweed soup, I can smell the aroma of the fresh seaweed. I tell myself this is what home smells like as I take a deep breath." In this sense, specific family foods were consecrated, cast as sacred objects, gifts of love. Most memories were awash in sentimentalism. Even in the cases of memories of otherwise unbearable family circumstances, food signified love and redemption. "I grew up in a home with my alcoholic mother . . . [W]hen I could smell bread baking, I knew it was a good day. On the rare occasion that she would not drink, I would come home to find a clean house and a loaf of bread in the bread maker."[39]

While specific foods served as symbols of family identity, the shared act of eating was recognized as playing an important unifying role for family members. In this way, the family meal works as "a symbolic cultural anchor," to borrow phrasing from Hochschild—idealized, for many of these young people, as a site to resolve conflict, as one writer so tellingly wrote of "Sunday dinner where everything gets fixed."[40] While a few writers addressed ongoing family conflict—"Family dinners at my house are largely impersonal and should they get personal, it usually ends in an argument"[41]—the majority of young people idealized the family meal as a space to suspend conflict, holding at bay the excess demands and burdens that lay just beyond the family meal. Referencing brunch after church, one writer characterized the shared meal as a "safe haven from the rest of the week."[42] Consider this young writer: "We'd always sit down at the table as a family, putting work and other things aside to eat dinner together."[43]

When Daily Life Intervenes

Yet despite the symbolic importance assigned to them, shared meals were rarely discussed as routine events.

> Since I was little, I can hardly recall a time when my immediate family and I sat down at our dinner table and ate together. Most of the time because of my parents' work schedules and our after-school activities, it simply was not possible for us to eat at the same time. I know eating dinner together is good for children as they grow up and allows families to spend time together but that is not something we have ever been able to do realistically.[44]

When meal times were regularly shared, they were noted as a *cultural* exception, that is, something that happened in their families but that was uncommon in most other American families. For most, the family meal was reserved for special occasions, shared maybe once a week, sometimes once a year. Many family researchers have noted the time compression families face today such that time spent together must be negotiated.[45] In modern life, the family meal, wherein everyone eats the same food, at the same time, and in the same place, is hard won, cherished because it is so infrequent. As I listened to the interviews and read through the written narratives, I concluded that from the standpoint of young people, when it comes to food, families are barely muddling through. They made repeated reference to "busy schedules";[46] "schedules so packed";[47] "My parents were always busy and worked late";[48] "hectic schedules";[49] "My parents' schedules are very demanding, we barely sat down together."[50] This was often echoed in the interviews. "We try to eat together, like most of the time it doesn't, 'cause we're busy, so it doesn't really like work out," offered Lauren, a senior at a suburban high school, during her interview. In another interview, Allison, also a senior headed for college in the fall, whose parents are divorced and mother is remarried, offered with little affect, "We don't eat together," paused for a moment and then added, "My mom used to, she would make dinner every single night and now we have my step-dad and my step-brothers, we're all so busy, every once in a while we'll eat together. . . . I'm just involved in a lot of stuff." Changes in family form often alter family routines, as was well reflected in these young people's accounts.

Some identified concerted efforts to protect the sanctity of the family meal: "At dinner, TV's off, no phones. It's a form of respect," Janice, a sophomore in high school, explains during an interview. Kristen, a college sophomore, offers, "We would always wait for my dad to get home . . . [L]ike the TV wasn't allowed on." Youth identified "effort to preserve closeness together."[51] "We all had busy lives and lots of things to do but we always managed to find time every Tuesday night to get together."[52] Another writer riffs on a similar theme:

> My father's night off was Tuesdays, the only night that the four of us could have dinner together. My mom always made something delicious on those nights. My favorite dish was spaghetti with meat sauce. It was a dish the whole family can help with, which allowed for family bonding time. My father was in charge of toasting the garlic bread, my brother would set the table and fill the drinks, and I would prepare the salad and scoop the spaghetti noodles into everyone's plates. Sometimes our dinner would go on for two hours. These memories are especially precious to me now that we rarely eat together. When my mom makes spaghetti, my brother and I reheat it. Eating alone is not as fun as eating with family.[53]

Jennifer, a high school student from Washington High School, where I observed in the cafeteria, similarly explained in an interview, "On weekends, that's when we're actually together as a family, but weeknights are hard." Likewise, Becky, now a college student, said, "Growing up we didn't eat as a family since my dad was active duty, was always deployed, so it was like the three of us, my brother, my mom and I."[54] Becky explained that the three tried to eat together but that "sometimes things got busy or she'd [her mom] be gone and then it was like fend for yourself and that's when the microwaveable meals came out." "We would rarely sit at the table and eat because my father, sister and I would get home at different times. Usually we would eat our food in front of the TV in three different rooms," offered another writer.[55]

Many noted changing rhythms within their own families. "We *used* to live a somewhat parallel life to the Cleavers," one writer mused.[56] "I have many family food memories with my family, but few memories from my teenage years involve the whole family sitting down for a full meal together. Those scarce nights usually involved sitting down to a meal prepared solely by my mother and turning on the 5 o'clock news."[57] Young people remarked on life-course changes and the changing roles and obligations performed by family members, notably mothers, as families grew and adapted to shifting circumstances, often beyond their immediate control.

> I was young and my parents had just split up. My mom was working two jobs to put a roof over my sister's and my head, needless to say she didn't have very much money. She made this covered baked potato because it was inexpensive and tasted good. My sister and I thought it was a treat to have that meal and for a long time continued to think that. It is like a comfort food.[58]

Youth who belonged to immigrant families with origins outside the United States were more likely to write about shared meal times as a regular event and were also more likely to write about time spent with extended kin centered on food. Recall the earlier reference to the U.S. Census's finding that foreign-born families were more likely to participate in shared meals. I read many tales of immigrant families eating together, with high value placed on doing so. These two examples reflect a larger pattern taken from the whole.

> Being 100% Filipino, family and food are probably the biggest and best part of our culture. We have many get togethers, whether there is a special occasion or not. We take pride in our family and family comes first. . . . My mother and my aunts love to cook for our family; it's their favorite pastime. It was almost as if they did not believe in fast food, they were almost against it.[59]

> I have a huge family here and we all get together at least once a month at someone's house. I am from India so every time we have a get together, all we have is Indian food. . . . Those are the moments I cherish my whole life.[60]

But immigrant youth also talked about families in transition, moving away from extended kin and changing work commitments of adult family members: "I see my cousins as my brothers and sisters. There was a period of time where we all lived under the same roof. We would all sit together and enjoy my aunt's food. I think my favorite meal was *pasteles*."[61] But much had changed for this young writer; eventually he and his mother had moved into their own place in an adjacent town. Most immigrant youth writers talked about the careful balance required to maintain their family's distinct cultural foodways against the pull of the ease and convenience of American food practices. American food was largely taken to mean highly processed fast foods.[62] A few immigrant youth defined American enculturation in terms of the loss of the family meal as a shared cultural event and a drift toward commercially processed foods.

> My family came to America as refugees from Somalia . . . [I]t was difficult to adjust to our new life. At the time we dealt with this by talking it over at dinner every night with each other as a family. This was the routine for five years then things started to change. We eventually started to really like some of the American food such as pizza and hamburgers. My mom would still continue to cook but soon realized no one really wanted her food anymore. Family talks and cultural food for dinner turned into pizza while watching MTV. My mom says it still bothers her but we really haven't made an effort to change because this new living style is much more convenient.[63]

Evidence of change abounded in the narratives provided by these young writers. Fathers lost jobs; sometimes they thus moved out of the area in search of greater economic opportunity; parents divorced; mothers returned to work as their children grew older; new children were added to the unit; and parents had aging parents themselves to care for. As children grew older, they too faced an expanding array of outside obligations.

> As children, my sister and I were very active. Almost every night one of us was being whisked away to another rehearsal or practice. This made it very difficult to sit down and have dinner as a family every night. It *became* normal for my mother to cook dinner and we would all serve ourselves when we returned home from whatever it was we were doing.[64]

We had a hard time finding time to sit down as a family and eat, especially as my sisters and I got into high school—too many extra-curricular activities.[65]

I participated in many sports and other activities that kept our schedule extremely hectic. The easiest thing to do was snack or make what you can on your own. Often times we would eat out just because it was more convenient.[66]

By and large, family arrangements of the past were depicted longingly, and in direct contrast to family arrangements of the present. The recurring theme of longing for belonging persisted across both written narratives and interviews, as is illustrated in the case of this young writer.

I do not hesitate when I say my family is more than a little dysfunctional. On top of the recent addition of what some call the "second set" of my parents' children (my two youngest brothers 6 and 7), my father owns a restaurant, hotel, night club and is a co-owner of a Century 21 real estate company. My mother, while not being a taxi-driver for my three brothers, is an agent at Century 21. On a positive side, it hasn't always been this way. . . . Ten or more years ago it was just my dad, mom, my brother and I. My mom stayed home most of the time.[67]

Another offered, "I remember our family used to eat together at the table. This enforced table whittled away in the lives of our family. Where dinner used to be about family talk, it is now TV or nothing at all."[68]

For a small but significant number of writers, time was spent at home, just not together. These cases represented fractured families, physically together but emotionally alone. "Everyone's kind of doing their own thing," Jess explained in an interview. "I can't recall us ever sharing a meal together. Someone would cook in my family and people would grab a plate of food and head to their room, close the door and go about their business. Even during the holidays when everyone was home, we would NEVER sit together to eat. I always felt like no one ever really cared."[69] Another writer explained how this worked at home for her family:

We no longer eat food as a family. . . . Whenever lunch or dinner is ready to eat, we serve ourselves at the same time but we take our plates and either go to our rooms to use the computer while eating or sit in the TV room. . . . Each of us prefers to eat our own type of food. My brother likes fast-food types whereas I prefer to eat more healthy and cultural foods.[70]

Others echoed this theme: "We no longer eat as a family";[71] "My family and I don't eat a lot of meals together. My dad will cook and we will grab the food and either go upstairs or we will eat it at different times";[72] "We normally do not have everyone sit at the table because some people actually prefer to eat alone."[73]

Holiday Meals

A widespread perception of a decline in shared meal times helps to explain the special place holiday meals with extended kin assumed in youth's accounts. "I always looked forward to Thanksgiving because it was the only time I celebrated a holiday with a home-cooked meal. It's probably the best tasting food I'd eat all year since my diet consists mostly of fast food and repetitive meals."[74] His words were echoed in many narratives. "Growing up I was more-or-less on my own when it came to finding something to eat in my house. Really the only time cooking was a must was for Thanksgiving and Christmas," another writer explains.[75]

Holiday meals were typically conceived as an idealized sphere of family togetherness. Set against the daily family food routines, holiday meals from Thanksgiving to Dwali to Eid[76] and Christmas were "magnified moments" flooded by excesses of love, family togetherness, and an abundance of food.[77] "Food stretched beyond what the eye could see, family members packed in like sardines around a formal dining room table which was rarely used because there was junk covering it throughout the year."[78] "A house full of people and a lot of food."[79] Food is plentiful: "non-stop food";[80] "pumpkin pie, cherry pie, apple pie . . . five different kinds of cheesecake. . . . Three turkeys and two hams."[81] "We would have around 10 different dishes";[82] "We cooked as if there was no tomorrow";[83] "a house full of people";[84] "lots of food and fun";[85] "a house full of laughter, love, warmth and happiness";[86] "We always had many, many desserts and they were always homemade. We had things like pumpkin roll, chocolate sugar and pumpkin cookies, and pumpkin pie, shoo-fly pie, apple pie and much more."[87]

Historian Elizabeth Pleck suggests that sentimental domestic occasions, like holiday dinners, emerged in the mid-nineteenth century "as a solution to the social changes created by the industrial revolution . . . anxious by the growth of commerce and industry . . . Sentimental domestic occasions provided an orderly way of celebrating and made people feel more comfortable with modernity by reassuring them they were engaged in something truly old-fashioned."[88] In short, Pleck argues, the importance attached to holiday meals was a means to manage deepening middle-class anxieties about industrial expansion.

Today, the geographical dispersal of family members, owing in large part to work obligations, such that adult sisters and brothers, grandparents, and aunts and uncles are scattered across the map, contribute to greater investment in holiday meals over more routine meals to achieve the desired end of family togetherness. Even in the case of geographic closeness, time demands were such that family togetherness had to be sought in the cracks and cleavages of busy routines. "Thanksgiving," as one writer notes, "one of the best holidays for my family, is the only time where my parents and I can actually get a day off from work or school."[89] "During the year my family and I don't really get the opportunity to eat together as a family for dinner because of our different schedules. Someone is always busy or working so eating together as a family for Christmas and Thanksgiving means a lot."[90]

Thanksgiving, Chanukah, Christmas, Eid, and Diwali occupied an important place in the narratives precisely because these holidays provided something daily meals did not, that is, the momentary glimpse of a strong family core on which to hang hopes for greater family connection and a collective identity to anchor the self.[91] Unlike the daily meal, characterized by many writers as a free-for-all, where everyone fends for himself or herself, at the holiday meal the collective trumps the individual.

Motherly Love, Processed Foods, and Home-Made Pie

Just as holiday meals emerged as symbolic anchors of a strong family core, so did mothers, who were cast as important caretakers who through their love willed the family "we" into being. "The symbolic weight of the family is condensed and consolidated . . . increasingly now into the mother," Hochschild explains. The transformation of intimacy and family care brought by large-scale economic transformation has recast mothers into new symbolic roles. "The more shaky things outside the family seem, the more we seem to need to believe in an unshakable family and failing that, an unshakable figure of mother-wife."[92] Consider this account as illustration: "Every afternoon when my brother, sister and I got home from school, there would be a plate full of warm cookies along with a smile and a hug from my mother. . . . It was not the cookie though, it was the dedication that my mother had in the making of them each day."[93]

No doubt many readers already observed the prominent place of mothers in the narratives discussed thus far. Mothers' continued responsibility for primary caregiving is evident across the interviews and written memories. "My mother made it a point to eat dinner together as a family while growing up," offered one writer.[94] That mothers still maintain the bulk of obligation to provide family care is a well-substantiated claim supported by decades of careful research. Yet as obvious as its persistence is, it is also taken for granted, often passing easily without comment. What I found especially compelling about the narratives was not that mother's care was assumed but what mother's cooking meant to these young people. Mothers who cooked were mothers who loved. "[She] showed her love by feeding us," offered one writer.[95] The link between "mother love" and "home cooking" is enduring in the social imaginary, a yardstick against which children measure the depth of their mother's love.[96] I came to appreciate this fact one afternoon while talking with a mother as she told me how her daughter, now grown, had recently remarked to her how meaningful it was that she had prepared lunch and packed it in a brown bag every day of high school, while most other kids bought school lunch. Her lunch brought from home was taken as evidence of being cared for. But this is an expression of the enduring, though no less arbitrary, divide between the public and private provisioning of food, whereby the assumption is that only home-cooked food is bound to meanings of care, and food provided by public institutions, such as school lunch, is characterized in terms of indifference and the absence of care. In reality, a large number of parents depend upon a public food-provisioning system to provide this care. In 2013, twenty-one million children received free or reduced lunch as part of the National

School Lunch Program.[97] Lots of parents have their children buy school lunch because they are busy with other family and work demands, yet other parents eventually permit their children to buy lunch after successive lobbying attempts by children themselves to convince their parents to let them.

Despite this more complex reality, a moral divide persists whereby the home-cooked meal is cast against the encroachment of commercial and institutional food stuff—one profane, the other sacred. One writer explained, referring to her mother, "She always would take time to make full course meals when I was younger. Healthy was what my mom aimed for and would never think about serving me and my dad McDonald's or Taco Bell for dinner."[98] Consider the telling words of another writer: "When I reminded my mom the other day about the TV dinners [eaten when younger because the mother had a midnight shift as a police officer], she barely remembered. She told me she must have pushed that bad memory out of her mind. For her, those were the worst of times, having to leave her young children for hours on end, without a home cooked meal."[99] That so many youth extolled this motherly virtue is probably a way to signal one's having been loved *and* evidence of belonging to a caring family unit as a whole.[100] "I love my mother's cooking. From a young age until I left for college my mom cooked a homemade meal almost every night of the week. She'd cook when she got home from work," another writer echoed.[101] When this motherly care is absent, family members inevitably turn to the commercial realm, but not without misgivings or dramatic transformation in the meaning of who they are as a family. For those whose mothers were unable or unwilling to provide home-prepared meals, a lingering tone of disappointment and loss prevailed.

When I was six, my mom told me that I wasn't going to be the only child anymore and that she was pregnant with my brother and sister (twins). She was always so tired so I started to help out more and make dinners. She started buying dinners in a box. The chicken cordon bleu with the side of hand-made rolls and butter became less and less until it was no more. Spaghetti-O's, macaroni and cheese, hot dogs, hot pockets and microwavable pizza now line my fridge. Twelve years later the only thing left of my mom's amazing cooking is the pumpkin pie she makes on Thanksgiving. She rolls the dough by hand and creates this crust that goes perfectly with pumpkin pie flavor.[102]

Social scientists have observed that many of the tasks once performed by wives or mothers in the home have been outsourced, increasingly provided by paid workers, rather than redistributed among family members. Many of the narratives spoke to this. "My mom only makes Filipino food and she is a great cook. If everyone is too lazy to cook food, which used to happen once every two weeks, my parents would buy fast food."[103]

Because home-cooked foods tended to carry greater moral weight than processed or store-bought meals, they were a means to make symbolic distinctions of value, and thus important to the symbolic and moral boundaries family members draw between families. "My cakes were homemade," one writer explained, remembering childhood birthdays proudly.[104] "Most children's favorite meals probably came out of a Happy Meal box but mine came straight from the ground," wrote Josh, a nineteen-year-old who went on to detail the harvesting of basil from his mother's garden to make pesto, his favorite meal.[105] Another writer, originally from the Ukraine, offered, "As I visit my friends I notice they have chips, soda, frozen foods and other kinds of fast-cooked foods. Neither I had those in Ukraine nor do I right now in America. My house never had any non-home cooked food or junk food."[106] Another echoed a similar theme: "We always ate home-cooked meals and I cannot remember eating a television dinner even once as a child."[107] It is noteworthy that in the last two cases, family origins reside outside the United States, the presumed epicenter of commercial, processed foods. Historian Simone Cinotto notes that eating out emerged as a popular leisure activity for U.S. families in the 1920s; the rising appeal and necessity of eating out advanced the public consumption of food, something we now take for granted as part of the everyday food landscape. As much as the commercial sphere is cast as anathema to family, the reality is that family making regularly unfolds in commercial settings, and is thus not antithetical to it.

As far as I can remember, all three meals at my house consisted of traditional Indian food. It did not take long for me to get tired of eating everything with *roti*. My parents always stressed that we had to maintain our cultural identity and that a good way to do this was to eat in a traditional Indian manner. My father sympathized with my sister and I and made the decision that every Saturday we would eat out. I still remember the first time I ate at Roy Rogers. . . . My whole family started looking forward to every Saturday.[108]

In some cases, even family traditions are made through commercial markets.

In my family when my brothers and I were younger it was a tradition that every Friday night was happy meal night. It was always a big treat. We would wait all week just to get the happy meals because it also meant we got a toy and were able to have soda that night. After school around 5ish, when our babysitter left, my mom would take us through the drive up at McDonald's to order our food. The tradition ended when I went to middle school because I was the youngest and by that time we all had different schedules. We have all said when we have kids we are going to carry this tradition on with our families.[109]

A number of young people shared memories of the McDonald's drive-through, or other such place, suggesting, as sociologist Viviana Zelizer has, that the commercial realm of market and the sentimental realm of family lack clear dividing lines. Like Zelizer, the anthropologist Dan Miller analyzes "consumption as a process of value creation" whereby individuals create "a sense of the inalienable through consumption"[110] and commodities are objectifications of relations of love and care.

McDonald's has been in the business of crafting memories through advertising campaigns for a long time, yet the memories young people narrated were often rooted in the actual activities of families themselves. "I eat at McDonald's," Allison explained. "My dad used to work there for a really, really long time. What I remember from being little is my dad working at McDonald's. My mom worked at Baskin Robbins so those are like comfort food for me. . . . McDonald's it just reminds me of when I was little." Consider these narratives as further examples:

My parents' schedules are very demanding, so we barely sat down together and ate a meal as a family. My mother would frequently cook, however, we would all eat at separate times depending on our schedule. The predominant memory I have of eating McDonald's every week is the feeling of family togetherness we had as a family each week when we sat together to eat. The food itself made no difference. The reason for McDonald's was it was easy, fast, and something we all enjoyed.[111]

My mom always got off work around 6 p.m. and my dad would always work late on Thursdays. So every Thursday my mom would have to pick my sister and I up from "extended" day care and we both knew what that meant—McDonald's! Since my mom did not feel like cooking after a long day at work, she would always take us to McDonald's and my sister and I would be ecstatic.[112]

Another writer, whose family migrated from India, offered, "Pizza is a must once a week and I can never forget Chipotle on Fridays. I do love those days because those are the times when I notice my mom, dad and brother eating with me together." He went on to explain that at home, "[I]n my family we usually don't sit together, my mom usually cooks food for us and serves it while we are eating. She eats last."[113] Here family ties, our most durable social bonds, are forged though face-to-face encounters in a commercial sphere. Importantly, the commercial realm frees up his mother to partake in shared eating. Sociologist Dan Cook presses the point: "Goods, brands and associated commercial meanings thereby figure directly into the shape of the emotional lives of children. . . . Children thus become part of the culture of consumption in large part through others who are acting as caring loved ones, tied to them, not through commodity logic but by threads of intimacy."[114] The profane world of economic interest embodied in fast-food outlets, store-bought meals, and heavily processed and packaged foods and the sacred realm of love embodied in the home-made meal are after all not so distinct as one often presumes.[115]

Remembering Food, Remembering Family

I have a confession to make. When I began this project, I was not much of a cook. My mother never really cooked herself, seeing it mostly as a source of domestic drudgery, even though she was home with us until I was in middle school. I never learned to cook from her; she actively discouraged any movement on the part of my sister and me into the kitchen, fearing we would then be forever tethered to it. As I got older my father began to cook more, but in high school I was too busy with other things to pay attention. In my twenties, I fumbled through the kitchen, cobbling together something resembling meals on the cheap. And then I married a man who genuinely enjoys cooking. He had learned his way around the kitchen from his mother. Though I cook now and enjoy it, my husband is still a much better cook than I am. He moves intuitively around the kitchen, whereas I adhere to recipes. Two things set in motion my interest in home cooking. The first had to do with this project. Reading through the written narratives and the interview transcripts over and over, it was difficult to ignore the fact that for these young people, mother's cooking was about love and care. I wanted my two daughters to have memories of their mother, and not just their dad, cooking home-made cookies and pies for them and with them. So out of a deep desire to occupy a special place in my children's memories, I began to cook. I suppose this is one of those examples of how our research projects shape us as much as we shape them.

The second reason why I began to cook has to do with the dilemmas of work-family balance. Many feminists in the 1970s abandoned the domestic slog of home in pursuit of rewarding work and personhood outside the home. But in an odd reversal, mothers today often feel strapped for time as the demands of work pull us away from family. Home is something we have less time for. Husbands and wives both report feeling overburdened with work. Feminists today are much more likely to talk about finding balance between the competing demands of work and family for women and men. As a university professor, at a public university where faculty have substantial research, teaching, and service commitments that often mean grading papers and answering e-mail into the late hours, long after children have gone to bed, where portions of Saturdays and Sundays are regularly forfeited to work, the act of cooking for and with my family has often felt like an effort to build symbolic walls to keep work out and to preserve our most durable ties of love. I'm not alone here. American adults continue to place tremendous importance on the family. Pew Research Center's social-trends data found that 76 percent of all adults report that family is the most important element in their life, even as they have less time to give to it.[116] This chapter suggests that children, many transitioning to adulthood, also place a very high value on family and would like to have more time for family centered in and around food, in and outside the home.

This chapter has sought to explore the symbolic currency of longing and belonging as young people talk about food and family life, examining the tension between family as a sphere of practical activity and family as a symbolic sphere of moral meaning. Both are shaped by processes of marketization that prevail in a period of late capitalism, creating tremendous time demands on children and their adult family members.[117] In this context, family meals come to occupy a precarious place.

Yet, there is some debate about the extent to which changes in the family meal are entirely new or instead reflect a misinformed nostalgia about what we think family meals used to represent. For eighteenth-century American families, Cinotto suggests, "The notion of the meal as a regular, structured activity of family life was at best vague."[118] She argues further, "The ideal of the proper family mealtime, originally devised by the Victorian middle class, gained cultural hegemony in modern America, but with the partial exception of the 1950s, only a minority of American families could ever live by it."[119] Husband and wife sociologists Robert and Helen Lynd's famous study of *Middletown,* based in the Muncie, Indiana, of the 1920s, noted family members being pulled away from evening meals by outside activities. Of "meal-time" they wrote, "under the decentralizing pull of a more highly diversified and organized leisure—in which basket-ball games, high school clubs, bridge clubs, civic clubs, and Men's League dinners each drain off their appropriate members from the family groups—there is arising a conscious effort to 'save meal-times, at least, for the family.'"[120] Historian Stephanie Koontz is also careful to remind us, "Families have always been in flux and often in crisis, they have never lived up to nostalgic notions about the way things used to be. But that doesn't mean the malaise and anxiety people feel about modern families are delusions."[121] So, what gives?

Arlie Hochschild's formulation of family life on a commercial frontier offers some explanation. Hochschild argues that the institutionalized dimensions of care have weakened, while a concurrent transformation, whereby "care has moved up in ideological importance, as part of an intense and hazy quest to create a kinder, gentler family and nation," has also taken shape.[122] As the cultural landscape of care transforms on the "commodity frontier," as Hochschild has called it, boundaries between home and market are increasingly blurred. The consequence, she argues, is a "hypersymbolized but structurally weakened core of the modern American family."[123]

Young people's increased obligations outside the home, combined with parental work obligations and the geographical dispersal of extended kin, impinge upon the collective act of eating as a family. Tricia, a student from Washington High School, explains, "I'm a three-sports athlete. So a lot of time after school I'll go to like Subway or McDonald's or Starbucks." As public rhetoric of care intensifies, the "practical realities" of everyday families often stand at odds. It is in this context that the family meal emerges as "a symbolic cultural anchor" for families' youngest members.[124]

However, memories are funny things. They are highly selective. It is in this sense that the question of memory must also be considered, and its precarious relationship to our actual everyday worlds and the events out of which it is made.[125] This, I think, is relevant in terms of the way we understand the relationship between changes to individual family routines and rituals resulting from life course changes as children edge toward adulthood, on one hand, and, on the other, historical transformations to the collective life of families as a societal whole.

Families change over the life course. Children grow older and more independent, their outside activities increase, parents change jobs. These life course changes that impact the dynamics of discrete family units, I suggest, are often made sense of through a lens of cultural nostalgia for a largely fictional collective past of family cohesion that is set against fractured families of the present—what Coontz referred to as the "families we never were."[126] At the same time, our cultural expectations of families and family time have intensified, as have our expectations of what children need from their parents. These are the ideas held by parents, but also by young people. Sociologists have found, on the basis of time-use diaries, that parents spend more time with their children today, not less, than they did in the 1960s, though mothers spend less time cooking.[127] This suggests that longing has much to do with our changing expectations of family care. The longing for the sense of family togetherness experienced in early childhood as children grow older and begin their transition into adulthood at a historical moment of increasing demands combines with broader cultural longings for family unity and cohesion held by young and old in the face of genuine cultural and economic changes to families that make family food provisioning much more difficult to do.

Our sentimentalism intensifies around food as relationships of intimacy and care shift in both the life and the social organization of individual families and the institution of family itself. Perhaps this should come as little surprise at a historical moment when "children live in their own separate world, which lacks connection to the past," explains Hochschild.[128] Home-based food remains a symbol of intimacy and care in what Charles Taylor has termed "the modern social imaginary"—that is, "how we collectively imagine" our social existence—which makes possible "common practice and a widely shared sense of legitimacy."[129] Home-based food in the social imaginary thus provides important clues about our collective longings, promising unity and wholeness at a time when the self is pulled in various directions and family members, young and old, manage a transforming set of obligations as they confront changes to public and private spheres of existence. Yet, this chapter also casts a long shadow on food provisioning in the home, revealing how very fraught food as a private good is and its current limits as families confront a broad array of constraints and must bend to the will of large-scale change. In the next chapter, I continue to explore the ties between food and care, not in the private realm of home and family but in the public institution of school, where food is a public good, examining the difficult work of bringing into being a public food-provisioning system, the contradictory role of commercial food markets, and the enduring force of social inequality in school.

2

The Cafeteria as Great Equalizer

Making Food Good

An electronic bell signals the end of one lunch period and the beginning of a new one. Overhead, I hear a syncopation of shuffling feet, laughter ricocheting off the walls of the wide halls that lead to the cafeteria, where I stand, waiting just beyond Thurgood High School's international food station, one of several stations where lunch can be bought each day by Thurgood's twenty-two-hundred-plus students. As the second lunch of the day gets underway, crooked lines rapidly take shape. Teens, almost all black and brown, many part of the "near-poor," dart in quick succession from the four corners of the room, much like pinballs, all in an effort to beat the rush. Others trickle in. Taking their time, they stroll at a casual pace. Unlike in the classroom, in the cafeteria you do not have to be in your seat before the second bell rings. In fact, you don't have to sit at all. The volume in the room begins its steady climb, and I watch as lunch erupts around me. Two girls bounce into one of the lunch lines; both purchase a ready-made Rice Krispies Treat and an individual package of Pop-Tarts before heading back into the hall from where they came. Another girl's stretched arms offer warm greeting to a missed friend; fists bump against each other as two boys, both dressed in the familiar sneakers, hoodies, and dark denim skinny jeans, stand just feet from the pizza line. The pizza line, always the longest, stretches out the door. Today's featured pizzas are vegetable and pepperoni. With the exception of the crust, I am told by Brenda, the school district food director, the pizza is made on site the same day it is served.

I stand idle, watching as kids, trays in hand, cycle in and out through the maze of tightly packed lunch stations. A boy yells out, "Yo! Jose," from his place in the grill line, another food station where (baked, not fried) french fries could be bought every single day of the school year last year, but as of this year, now only once a week. The station beside it, modeled after Manhattan Deli, a popular sandwich franchise, offers a selection of sub sandwiches. Its line is shorter than the grill and pizza lines, but appreciably longer than the almost nonexistent salad line, where students can purchase a ready-made salad. "Is this your lunch?" a boy calls out across the stations as he holds a tray with a low-fat milk, a small pile of grapes, chicken, and rice. "Ooohhh we are c-u-t-ting!" one girl, with rows of small braids stretching down her back, declares as she eyes the dense, noisy lines, snaked out the wide garage-like doorways of the food stations. Another girl declares, "Oh I'm not going to eat, forget this," as she turns on her heels and heads out toward the tables. A tall, leggy girl stands just beyond the line for pizza. Pleading with the boy beside her, she clasps his wrist with both hands, pulling him gently toward a shorter line; he does not budge and she eventually loosens her hold. Another girl announces assuredly to a boy walking by, "We are getting salad—salad is what we should get." She laughs after she says this and heads toward the pizza line. I don't see any kids get salad.

"What the—? This is bullshit," I hear a girl say, voice full of exasperated protest. Full-bodied with curly brown hair pulled into a messy high ponytail, she stands at the register, tray before her, hand on hip, a deep scowl across her face as she shakes her head emphatically. I realize she has been accused of not paying for her juice. She is adamant that she has as she shakes her head one more time, before she quickly pivots and walks out. With a quiet sigh, the lunch lady lets her go, turning her attention toward the boy next in line, and begins to tally the items on his tray. I see "$0.25" flash quickly on her computer screen, and I realize his is a reduced lunch. He pins his lunch code in an instant, grabs his tray, and heads out the door, passing a girl with an ample frame, dressed from head to toe in black, and a lanky boy, trailing inches behind her. They go through the line together and then he waits, just beyond the cash register. She punches in her pin, "$0.25" again flashes on the screen, and then she nonchalantly passes off to him the tray of food, which he takes, offering a perfunctory thanks and heading to another table where sit three girls, two of whom I had already seen in the previous lunch period. The girl heads in the opposite direction, toward one of booths that line the left side of the room, arriving at one where four other girls are already sitting. A large Utz chips bag sits on the table alongside an oversized Arizona Iced Tea bottle; neither has been opened.

Standing near the lunch line I am greeted by a tall, middle-aged white man, dressed in a light grey suit, who very nicely asks who I am and what I am doing. He is one of several vice principals at the school and is a permanent fixture of Thurgood's lunchroom. I explain my purpose, something to the effect that I am studying young people and food, which apparently sets him at ease, and he begins to remark on the food and what kids eat. Brenda, Thurgood's food director, a middle-aged white woman edging toward her sixties who has spent a lifetime in food service, has done "a lot" he tells me, in the eight years she has worked for the district. The school goes to great lengths to "make the food appealing to the kids," though he confides as he leans in toward me, "Yeah, but you *still* don't see kids eating fruits and vegetables." I nod along, though I had already seen several kids nibble on the grapes and baby carrots on their lunch trays as they wait in line. Our conversation ends abruptly as he spots two girls angling to cut the still-long pizza line. But his remark about "making the food appealing to the kids" stays with me. It is a point I return to again and again as I sift through the data I have collected for this project. What's involved in making school food appealing for kids? In many American public schools, making school food appealing to students remains a distant second to the all-important bottom line. Yet, in the other school I observed for this project, Washington High School, "making the food appealing" had also emerged as an important school district priority. Why? The aim of this chapter is to unpack the issue of school food's appeal and why it matters.

What kids eat in school and its impact on health outcomes have been subject to intense debate in the last decade, helping to make this an important public and policy matter. Across the political spectrum, we as a country accept on some level that schools play an important role in promoting the health and well-being of our children. Given that school is a public institution, nourishing the bodies and minds of students is its fundamental obligation. Yet, we often fall short. This can be explained partly by our ambivalence toward the public provisioning of food, an activity associated with caretaking in the intimate sphere of family and home. In the previous chapter, we were able to see how precarious the private provisioning of food is—how difficult it is for family members, as they navigate the outside pressure of work, children's changing schedules, and the growing complexity of family bonds, to get dinner on the table. And just as family life is shaped by the broader complex of social and economic forces, often too abstract to recognize its daily influence, so too is school. This chapter and the two that follow examine the complex of considerations involved in public food provisioning in school and the meaning of food as a public good. This chapter begins with a brief overview of school lunch over the last century, moving to a much fuller examination of the current state of school lunch as it is organized in one public high school. The chapter weaves together a set of divergent considerations that relate to public food-provisioning systems: how commercial food markets intervene and mediate school lunch; how disparities in and between schools pattern the type of food served; and how ideas about diet and health shape perspectives on food's appeal.

This chapter highlights the work of Brenda, the food director at Thurgood High School, with the aim to deepen our understanding of the complexity of school lunch as a high-stakes public good.[1] Another food director had introduced me to Brenda via e-mail about six months before I began observing at Thurgood. Brenda had a no-nonsense style about her; she rarely minced words, but was warm in her demeanor, knowledgeable, and accessible. Brenda made the best of what she was given but hoped for a better food future and in this sense was both pragmatic and aspirational. She held her ground in the face of outside scrutiny, and acknowledged the *social* value in her work and its link to a public system of care. She recognized that a larger number of students she fed each day were part of the growing number of those who are food insecure in the United States, and her effort to prepare food kids wanted to eat expressed a deep commitment to addressing both health and hunger.

One Hundred Years of School Lunch

Each morning school-aged children across the country leave their homes, some with breakfast in their bellies, others without, and head off to school. They venture beyond the world of home, out from under the umbrella of parental care. And by the start of the first bell, another group of adults, that is, teachers and school administrators, is responsible for them. While a core part of the care these adults provide is academic instruction, feeding is also an important component of the care schools provide to our children each day. While not without its struggles, the project of feeding children has been recognized as an important service schools, as public institutions, provide in pursuit of one of its most cherished ideals: equality of access and opportunity.

Schools have been feeding our children for just over a century. At the beginning of the twentieth century, PTAs, informed by the new science of nutrition and a moral imperative of caring for our youngest citizens, assumed the bulk of responsibility for the delivery of sound nutritional meals in school. This was done primarily in an effort to stave off poverty-related under-nutrition, and at the same time run an effective campaign to Americanize the large number of arriving immigrant children. "Hot lunches promised to protect America's youth from the scourge of malnutrition," the historian Susan Levine writes in her *School Lunch Politics*. "Healthy children, like public education more generally, signaled America's democratic strength."[2] Well-meaning PTAs and social reformers thought that school lunches, in addition to providing a well-balanced and nutritional meal, should also be educational to ensure a healthy citizenry.

It was not until the 1930s that school food became the policy matter it is today. From its policy beginnings, school lunch has been the subject of much debate, tied to the machinations of state and federal politics, shaped by an expanding commercial and industrial food market, and steeped in an emerging set of national commitments to the principles of rationalized governance and efficient organization, as well as the promise of both science and market-based strategies to resolve a host of social problems.[3] Levine's history of the rocky rise of the National School Lunch Program (NSLP) and its various iterations and transformations helps us to understand the political and economic complex under which school lunch for the last century has been organized. Levine reminds us that the struggle over lunch in the past reflected a much broader struggle over states' rights, and in particular southern states' efforts to thwart school desegregation, rather than the more straightforward matter of food and nutrition.

Markets and racial politics have long played a part in school lunch and continue to do so today. Debates over what role federal and state government should play in feeding our children and which children are most entitled to these government provisions have cast a long shadow over the twentieth century. Since its beginning, the NSLP, ratified in 1946, like lunchrooms themselves, bore the mark of racial segregation.[4] In the 1960s, estimates suggest that less than one-quarter of African American children were able to participate in the NSLP, while well over 50 percent of white children did.[5] Black children in the segregated South often attended schools that had no lunchroom facilities to provide lunch. Not all schools participated in the NSLP, even if they had students who would otherwise qualify for free or reduced lunch. Because state and local districts were left to administer the program on their own, there was considerable variance in its implementation. Levine reports that one city district required students to work for their "free" lunch.[6] In some quarters, school lunch programs were regarded as subversive and a site of contest over the fate of a nation. Conservatives of yesterday, just as they do today, raised a red flag, seeing federal overreach in local affairs and the communal institutional routine of mass feeding as a symptom of creeping socialism and weakened individualism, which run the risk of creating a generation of dependents, as Levine reports.

Today, we often think about NSLP as a program for kids in need. However, it was not initially conceived as a welfare program but instead as a program to feed all our nation's children, which it still does today. Only in the mid-1960s did the school lunch program emerge as a tool to address poverty and hunger, though its implementation lagged behind any congressional mandate until grassroots pressure forced the matter, increasing the number of poor children receiving free lunch in large numbers by the end of the 1960s, and giving rise to the New School Lunch Program Bill of Rights in 1969. As a program, it remains underutilized. Only 62 percent of those students who attend schools that participate in NSLP eat school lunch, according to the School Nutrition Dietary Assessment III.[7] It was not until several decades later, however, that the stigma of poverty, which has been associated with the NSLP since the late 1960s, has been reduced, though not eliminated by any stretch, by the use of student electronic pin numbers since all students pin in their personal identification number. It is more difficult when standing in line to determine who is paying out of their pocket and who is getting a free lunch. Meaningfully, it was not until 1994 that a congressional mandate required the USDA, which administers the NSLP, to be in compliance with the national dietary guidelines.[8]

School Lunch Today

It is probably no accident that the two schools whose food directors granted me access to the cafeteria for observation were schools that felt they had something to be proud of. Gaining access to a school cafeteria under scrutiny for its poor-quality food would, I suspect, have been much more difficult, if not entirely out of reach. Both, though in different ways, have been well ahead of the curve in terms of healthy food provisioning. Both Thurgood and Washington identified healthy food offerings as important district priorities, and the district food directors, Brenda and Dan, worked diligently toward that end. But the way each conceived of healthy food and student appeal differed significantly and was ultimately shaped by the student populations that the schools served. We are all well aware that some so-called healthy foods are quite delicious and others are not—that food tastes are at once highly individualistic and profoundly social in form. Our ideas about school foods' appeal are often difficult to disentangle from our assumptions about youth as a group, their tastes, what compels them to action, and how to get them to eat what we adults want them to eat.

These days school lunch is easy fodder. Discontent with school lunch offerings was a point that emerged in every single interview and focus group I conducted, irrespective of the high school attended. The extent to which school food fails in its appeal has been the subject of endless jokes. A visit to Facebook will reveal a slew of groups and community forums dedicated to chronicling how much "school lunch sucks." School lunch is often characterized as "gross" or "nasty" by kids from elementary school on up. And often it is, but not always. The fact that school lunch often is unappealing is bound up, as I have already suggested, with our cultural ambivalence about the *public* provisioning of food for children, an activity long associated with the private realm of home and motherly care. Arguably, characterizations of school lunch as gross or nasty are expressions of this ambivalence.

The prevailing assumption in many camps is that to make food appealing to kids requires a forfeit of health; kids will refuse the healthy offerings, generating enormous plate waste. But this is a questionable claim. While there certainly are kids content to eat pizza day in, day out, they do not represent the diversity of viewpoints held by young people about food. A recent study from UC–Berkeley's Center for Weight & Health found that a majority (69 percent) of high school students surveyed thought having fresh fruit on the menu more important than having chips, candy, or soda—quite the opposite of what we often think about teenagers' food preferences.[9] A majority of students surveyed also characterized their school food environments as unhealthy; most surveyed thought their schools should provide healthier food options than they did. In Janet Poppendieck's study, students also characterized their school food environment negatively; school food was usually described as "nasty," with students citing poor quality and lack of variety as chief reasons for disliking food.[10]

Without a doubt, food's appeal to youth is part of a larger calculus of concerns for food directors and the school districts that employ them, including labor, budget, constraints of both market offerings and the USDA's surplus food commodities program, federal nutritional guidelines, and the curricular aims of nutrition education. Making food appealing is hardly a straightforward proposition. High school cafeterias are spaces where multiple lines of social action collide, fomenting a push and pull that indelibly shapes the work of food directors.

Commercial food companies are major players shaping the public provisioning of food in school. The heavy dose of marketing by food and beverage industries has been, until very recently, part of the taken-for-granted backdrop of school lunch. With the exception of small, community-based groups of concerned parents, honest brokers like the Center for Science in the Public Interest,[11] and watchdog groups like Campaign for a Commercial-Free Childhood[12] or Corporate Accountability International,[13] the presence of McDonald's, Taco Bell, Sodexo, Coca-Cola, and Subway has hardly raised an eyebrow—nor has the fact that the food and beverage industry spends millions of dollars yearly to advance corporate interests by expanding corporate reach in school, too often at the expense of sound nutritional health for children. Schools have long faced a double bind because state funding for school lunches is typically insufficient to cover operational costs. As a case in point, Brenda was usually left with $1.10 per meal to meet federal dietary guidelines since about 40 percent of the federal reimbursement was absorbed by overhead costs. And thus, school food directors must find other means to generate revenues to stay afloat during the year.[14]

But as much as there are broad socio-historical trends to be noted in understanding the social organization of school food as a public good, there is also a deeply local character to the way schools manage the feeding of those in its care and craft lunch menus for youth appeal. Whether a school succeeds in serving healthy foods or forfeits to the reign of junk food depends on a complex set of both local and extra-local forces, what sociologists refer to as meso- and micro-level dynamics, as much as it does macro-level ones, such as broader food and educational policy, the reach of agribusiness and industry lobbies, or market deregulation. As Brenda herself admitted, perhaps somewhat defensively, "Every district in this country is different. They have different unique needs, different budgets."

Food Courts, School Cafeterias, and Commercial Markets

Thurgood High School is located among affluent suburbs of Washington, D.C., but a large base of students is bused in from the district's periphery, where lower-income and subsidized housing is concentrated. Nearly 60 percent of students receive free or reduced lunch, in comparison to less than 8 percent at Washington.[15] Many students at Thurgood belong to families who have been identified as "food insecure."[16] Thurgood is eligible for Title I resources, but does not accept them.[17] Thus, while Thurgood has worked to expand healthy options and improve healthy eating practices among its students, it also must address the issue of hunger. Thurgood is a large school, enrolling twenty-two hundred students in grades ten to twelve, and is ethnically and racially diverse, with 43 percent of the students being African American, 27 percent Hispanic, 21 percent white, 7 percent Asian/Pacific Islander and American Indian, and a large number of immigrants.[18]

Officially, Thurgood is a closed campus, which means that students are not permitted to leave school grounds during school hours, including lunch. Thurgood used to be an open campus. In the old school building, the cafeteria wasn't large enough to accommodate all students. The school had little choice but to allow students to purchase and eat lunch elsewhere. In essence, kids were farmed out to McDonald's and other places nearby, and in this way, school lunch was outsourced. Some kids went home for lunch. At the old school, the kids who ate in were mostly kids on free or reduced lunch, and thus eating in carried with it some element of poverty stigma.[19] Now that the campus is closed, nearly all stay for lunch. Of course, this doesn't mean kids don't leave campus. Occasionally, I stopped in at the McDonald's down the street after observing and was greeted by kids cutting school. I also witnessed kids sneaking out of school. One afternoon, I watched a vice principal chase after a group of boys who tore into a full sprint once they realized they were being tailed. After a full block, the vice principal gave up and returned to campus; the boys disappeared into the distance. Whether they returned to school that day, I can't say; but I did learn that administrators closed the campus when they moved to the new building three years previously in large part because of the chronic absenteeism that followed lunch for far too many students.

Thurgood's cafeteria is the centerpiece of the new building. Large enough to accommodate the swelling student population, it is a sprawling, open gathering place for the school; sunlight penetrates from skylights in the vaulted ceiling, making the room spacious and bright. The room is painted in school colors, promoting school unity and pride, and large black-and-white photographs depicting school events from an earlier era hang from its walls. As Brenda described, "We wanted it to be when people walked in they went, 'Wow!' I have taken so many groups through . . . [T]he first word out of their mouth is, 'This looks like a food court.'" In fact, it does look like a food court straight out of a scene from a shopping mall, with several food stations for pizza, burritos, sandwiches, salads, and burgers. With its focus on consumer choice with twenty entrée choices each day, self-service, and open seating, Thurgood's cafeteria is an example of the way commercial markets' influence in educational settings is a feature of American schooling in the twenty-first century.[20] To better tap student appeal and maximize student participation, food directors often turn to commercial food markets as guides. It is not uncommon that they develop a branding concept or follow trend profiles in taste, just as Brenda has. The fact of the matter is that school cafeterias have little choice but to compete against commercial outlets for students' money and loyalty, especially if they are an open campus where students can leave for lunch.

To say that teenagers' lives, inside and outside of school, are fully immersed in commercial markets is to state the obvious. One consequence of this, however, for schools is that commercial equivalents, whether one is talking about burritos, the salad bar, chicken nuggets, or Chinese food, are *the* yardstick for evaluation of school food. Whereas food in school cafeterias was supposed to at one point approximate home-cooked meals, the expectation today is that school cafeteria food is supposed to taste and look like commercial fast food. Nearly every young person I interviewed suggested that commercial counterparts were the primary reference in evaluating school lunch. "It's like the Chick-fil-A burger. It's like a knock off," seventeen-year-old Julie offered, describing the hamburger at her school. Jorge, a student at Thurgood, said much the same: "Friday they would have this like fake Chipotle, where they would pretend it was Chipotle, but it wasn't." Like Jorge, many students are unforgiving in their characterization of their school's failure to match up to its commercial counterparts.

That young people assess school food in relation to commercial fast food is hardly surprising given that the percentage of calories eaten away from home has increased substantially for children across age groups over the last quarter-century, transforming the categories we use to think about and evaluate food.[21] Many high schools, including Thurgood and Washington, are but a short walk from a cluster of commercial food settings, including McDonald's, Starbucks, and large grocery stores chains, allowing easy access to retail food outlets, even if the school is an officially closed campus.[22] I frequently observed students congregating at the McDonald's by Thurgood after school, just as I observed students in a food outlet a stone's throw away from many a suburban public high school. Even if kids aren't there in large numbers during school hours, they certainly are after hours.

Well aware that this is the reality in which food directors operate today, Brenda worked with students and administrators to improve the appeal of both the cafeteria space and its food offerings, promoting the cafeteria as an inclusive space, all the while "maintaining nutritional integrity within the budget." How did she do this? Adopting tactics from a marketing playbook, she enlisted the students to conduct and participate in focus groups and student-generated surveys, conducting what is essentially market research, to find out what kids wanted in a cafeteria, what they ate, where they ate, and how much they wanted to spend. What did she learn? Kids wanted a cafeteria that didn't feel like school.

"They didn't want it to be too academic," Brenda told me. "They didn't want to feel like they were in school when they came into the cafeteria." In fact, it doesn't feel like school at all, especially when compared to the many other cafeterias I have visited.

The cafeteria was intentionally designed to maximize appeal to counter the problems of low participation, all the while keeping health in the foreground. But as Brenda put it, "It's not cheap to do healthy." In fact, when they switched over to 100 percent whole wheat bread three years ago, it cost an additional seventy-five thousand dollars from an already burdened budget. In an effort to reduce processed foods, ones Brenda admits they rely on, they do much of the cooking on site.[23] Because they are tight on labor, a full round of scratch cooking is impossible since they get no school-board-budgeted funds. "There's no local tax dollars that come to our program. Sixty-three percent of my budget for revenue stream is from federal reimbursement," Brenda explained, which means they must be "very good stewards of our pennies."

Thus, it is within a set of pretty hefty budget constraints that they work to offer "fresh fruits and vegetables, whole grain items, and lower fat items," plan the menu around the "U.S. school challenge gold standard," and follow market trends on flavor profiles in order to appease students who want "good food . . . that's familiar to them." And while a large number of kids opt for pizza most days, kids ate beef tacos, bean burritos, Asian barbeque, chicken and rice, chicken fajitas, and black bean casserole. The food service staff also experiment with the menu, as Brenda explained.

> The international line, we decided that's going to be our experimental line. We'll throw everything on there from spaghetti to curry. . . . Today we had Brussels sprouts; that's new this year. . . . We try to stay up with the current trends. Asian is hot right now. So you kind of try to come up with those items and come up with in your budget some items that you might be able to throw out there that would, you know, appeal to the kids.

Since boredom with food is a central point of complaint by students, they regularly try out different possibilities, even offering sushi, as a "niche item" on the à la carte menu at five dollars a pop for kids willing and able to pay. "We have to kind of be a little bit creative with that.

What I think we do well is plain and simple food," Brenda explained. "You know, it's not the Ritz Carlton. . . . We also cannot necessarily be leaders in trends in the food market because of the fast-food industry, the quick-serve industry where kids eat a lot." As Brenda's remarks testify, schools face a sea of constraint that commercial food markets more easily avoid.

"The Great Equalizer": Markets and Moral Ends

Brenda's yielding to market models can certainly be understood as an example of the commercial food market's reach and influence. But ultimately this tells only half the story. A larger calculus of moral and public health concerns was also in play, reminding us of the complicated relationships among the various dimensions of our social existence and markets, the pull of privatization of public institutions, and the contradictions of market-based solutions to public problems. Her words often suggested a genuine concern for children's rights, as well as an awareness of the links between income inequalities and health disparities, suggesting that a food-provisioning system in school is inseparable from the public and collective obligation of care for children.

Decisions made in the market are rarely inspired by moral commitments, but at Thurgood that is not the case. Instead, the commercial market, its logic and its language, was a means to an end. As Rebekah Massengill noted in *Wal-Mart Wars*, "[P]eople and societies use markets to negotiate moral meanings and obligations."[24] This can be seen in Brenda's overvaluing of "consumer choice" and her characterization of "students as consumers." This language is increasingly used in educational settings, much to the dismay of many educators who see this as an example of corporate steamrolling of a core public institution upon which the civil sphere depends. "Some people will say, 'Well, these are students, they're not customers,'" Brenda explains. "They *are* customers. In my mind they are customers. They don't have to eat with us. We treat them like students . . . but we give them respect and I think it makes no difference what you call them. The point of it is that you respect everybody." While some might be critical of her language of "students as customers," her words reveal the complex interplay of markets, moral boundaries, the drift toward privatization, and the discourse of public goods shaping educational policy and practice today. The idea of "choice" is a convoluted concept, as Brenda suggests. On the one hand, it is mediated by market ideas about consumer choice; on the other hand, "choice" is also part of a broader public discourse and an emerging set of modern attitudes about children's rights that encompass protections against harm and basic entitlements to care. Respect, a symbolic good gifted to consumers and thought to reside in the consumer sphere, like "choice," remains elusive for students. It is the case that students, especially those who are poor, move through school without the basic dignities and respect extended to others.[25] Her words about "respect" of the student consumer assume additional significance as she worked to improve the way food service workers ("the lunch ladies") treated the kids, after outside observers remarked to her, "Your staff isn't friendly." This was also a point of complaint by some students.

> Oh my god . . . I won't even say anything to the lunch ladies other than "Hi, how are you?" . . . [T]here were some that were really patient but others were completely rude, like rude with everybody. And just because some kid says something to them or does something to them or because they steal something, they would take it out on everybody that came in the line.

Another young woman echoed her remarks: "I would get really mad and frustrated because they would like yell at me for something that I didn't do." Undoubtedly, this is a complicated issue and is certainly not specific to Thurgood. Respect, demanded by teachers and administrative staff, is often denied to food service workers, because they are low-wage workers whose jobs have been deskilled. Like many students, they labor under circumstances where dignity is denied. Their adult status is often the only status claim they can reasonably assert.

As paradoxical as a focus on "students as consumers" may be, since it serves to further embed a market logic in school, thereby collapsing citizen and consumer, it also lays the grounds for students' voices, often silenced or ignored, to get heard.[26] That students were entitled to basic rights of care and respect was also expressed in Brenda's contrast between the new cafeteria and the old: "[A]t the old school the cafeteria was in the basement and the chairs and tables were kind of ratty looking . . . [I]t was like a dungeon. . . . It was horrible, no light, nothing." While the old cafeteria was institutional, "dark and dreary," a symbol of an underfunded public provisioning system, this new space, a revitalized public space, modeled after the privatized commercial setting of a shopping mall food court, communicated student value and recognition. As Brenda remarked of "[t]he first kids that ever got to come into the [cafeteria]," "I'll never forget those kids. They came through and said, 'Wow, they thought that much of us to make this building,'" adding, "The kids were really appreciative."

This took on special significance since so many of the students are low income and without access to resource-rich schools. Many educational scholars have noted the decrepit conditions of schools that serve poor students: broken windows and doors, clogged toilets, books missing pages, computers that barely work, mold, leaky faucets, and peeling paint remain fixtures of these schools.[27] Thurgood looked nothing like one of those schools, and many at Thurgood worked diligently to keep it that way.

For Brenda, school food belonged to a moral sphere of action where a public health agenda was aligned with a public education agenda and was rooted in a commitment to public care. "I wouldn't be here if I didn't care and care deeply." This is the reason why Brenda is more than a little indignant about the increasing scrutiny food directors face in the public eye. Feeling much maligned, Brenda offered, "It really offends me when people are ill informed and just say, 'You know, you should do all fresh cooking.' It can be done in certain places. But you still have to work incrementally to make change and unfortunately people don't always want to see that. . . . It's hard work and it's worthwhile work." Motivated by a set of both pragmatic and moral concerns centered on maximizing access to healthy foods for a student population whose access to healthy foods outside school was thought to be severely limited, Brenda saw food as a vehicle to address persistent inequalities and poverty for students and their families. There was widespread acknowledgment among the staff and administrators that for some kids, their only meals were at school. "We know that we've got kids that only eat here," Brenda confided.[28]

Brenda worried that if the kids didn't have a range of food offerings, they might go without food or, just as bad, reject what was offered and opt for something with much lower nutritional value than what she served. This was one among several reasons why Brenda found herself critical of the emerging "chef's movement" (a movement to improve school food spearheaded by Ann Cooper of Berkeley's Unified School District in Northern California) and some of its guiding philosophies, especially the argument that "kids, if they're hungry, will eat what you give them if it's fresh and healthy." Brenda explained her thinking on the matter: "[W]hen they're [chefs] in schools they will offer one entrée. I just can't wrap around that because I'm thinking, 'Okay, I offer let's just say, a burrito and we've handmade it. We made everything from scratch. . . . What happens to the kids who don't like burritos? Do they just not eat that day? Or if it is a beef burrito being served, what about the vegetarians? "If I'm feeding twelve out of a hundred, I'm not doing my job," Brenda opined. Some schools have participation rates well below 15 percent, she remarked indignantly, seeing this as a failure of schools in "meeting our promise," by which she means schools' public mandate of equal access to care for those in their charge. Brenda often invoked this kind of moral language as she spoke about the responsibilities she and the school itself carried. For Brenda, it was important to "give kids options, to get them to experiment with foods, to try new foods, and to try to educate them about foods."

Observing students as they ate lunch, I was hard pressed to find reasons to be critical of Brenda and her approach. In my observations, very few kids openly complained about the food and not because they just weren't eating it. I overheard few if any characterizations of school lunch as "gross" or "nasty"; complaints were hardly the prevailing perspective held by kids.[29] The most common complaint at Thurgood was the long lunch lines. More than anything else, kids expressed boredom with food, but I often wondered if that really expressed their boredom with school. Sure, the handful of kids I interviewed from Thurgood called for "more variety" in the food, "more variety of fruits," "healthier stuff," "more salad options." "You eventually get bored with the same things, the salads never change," offered one student. "When you're trying to go healthy you're basically stuck eating salads . . . I actually did that for like a month but after that I couldn't do it," explained another Thurgood student. But other students thought highly of the cafeteria at Thurgood, characterizing it as a "great cafeteria . . . [O]ther schools I've seen their menu and it's awful." Another student noted, "A lot of people complain about Thurgood, but it's not so bad." I suppose there is the possibility that because kids expect school food to be gross, it being gross fails to warrant comment, but at Thurgood, I saw the vast majority eating what was offered. There was very little in the way of plate waste.[30]

Comments from Thurgood students contrasted with interviews with students from other schools, who regularly complained about their food. "The pizza is really disgusting. You had to blot the grease off the pizza," explained Clarisa, who attended high school in another school district. "We have grape fights 'cause the grapes they gave us were frozen. Nobody wants to eat them . . . so we just throw them." Alicia, who attends school with Clarisa, elaborates: "The strawberries suck, the lettuce is dry. . . . Nobody likes the mac and cheese . . . [S]ome of the people say it tastes like throw up." One student, also from another school district, who rarely bought lunch, described school lunch as "two things of French fries, a couple of cookies and maybe a main dish. They'll eat everything else and maybe take two bites of the main dish and then throw it away." Judy explained why she brings lunch from home and opts to not buy school lunch. "I don't really think it's that healthy . . . [I]t's like having fast food throughout the week. It's kind of like eating Mc-Donald's every day." Lauren, from another high school, described lunch as "French fries every day, pizza everyday . . . and then they'll have like rotten fruit. Nothing is fresh." With some histrionics, Sara described lunch as "[h]orrible. Not even close to food. It could be crawling off your plate at any second . . . fake cheese, fake bread," "[t]hree-day old chicken," "[a]wkward tuna." Setting the melodrama aside, her characterization captures the perception of school food held by many public school students. While some of these complaints can be explained by boredom with limited food offerings, the lack of food choices—"I just wish it was more do-it-yourself and I think that would have healthier choices"—their words also speak to considerations of nutritional health and freshness.

Brenda was confident that her meals exceeded nutritional requirements, and she had the data to prove it. Each year she would analyze the food kids brought from home and consistently found school meals more nutritious. UC–Berkeley's Center for Weight & Health also found that students who participated in the NSLP were more than twice as likely to consume fruits and vegetables, suggesting that the widespread perception of school lunch as a failing public project deserves reevaluation and perhaps reflects our inclinations to assume that public institutions and their services are inferior to the services provided by private industry. Brenda often made reference to empirical studies as a legitimate basis for her nutritional decisions: "I try to be an evidence-based program rather than a philosophy of eating. I try to think about the science of eating," she explained, and this is why she found herself critical of the chef's movement and the food reforms that were rooted in "a food philosophy" as opposed to science, seeing them as largely concerned with the aesthetics of food more than with public health.[31] This came to the fore over the matter of flavored milk, which has been the subject of contentious debate in many school districts, including Washington, D.C., public schools. Following the passing of the 2010 D.C. Healthy Schools Act, flavored milks had been eliminated from school lunch in an effort to reduce sugar consumption. Brenda professed her reservations about such a move, despite increasing pressure from the PTA in her own district.

> People say, "Well, if you just take it away from them they'll just drink the white milk." That's just not absolutely consistent with the research. Even in districts where chefs have been, they have gone back to flavored milks. That's what kids will drink.[32] What's wrong with flavored milk? . . . I will argue to the death. . . . I guess I don't care if there's three teaspoons of sugar in chocolate milk or strawberry milk. What I care is that the kids drink eight ounces of milk and get nine nutrients from that milk. I can't replace that any time else during the day. I can't replace magnesium, the phosphorus, the calcium. If they want to eat broccoli, fine, but it's going to take them a pound of broccoli to equal that.[33]

Brenda was assiduous in her efforts to provide nutritious meals that kids would eat. The stakes for Brenda, I came to realize, were especially high. For one thing, there was an economic obligation to maximize student participation to avert budget shortfalls. But she also was compelled to maximize student participation lest the cafeteria revert back to what it once was, a place where only poor kids eat. Brenda was mindful of the stigma associated with poverty and hunger and felt reasonably confident that her cafeteria had successfully addressed the stigma associated with free and reduced lunch. Referring to the now widely used electronic pin system that students use to purchase lunch, she explained, "I think that's one of the best things we've ever done for kids . . . [T]here's no stigma. As they go through the line, they put in their number . . . [N]obody knows they are free reduced." While it is not entirely true that poor kids escape detection by others, the newer electronic pin system used by all students has reduced the visible markers identifying one's status as reduced-lunch-eligible. Now, school lunch can be purchased more easily without the worry of being (whether correctly or incorrectly) "outed" as poor.[34]

Providing niche items like sushi also prevented defection by those kids who could easily afford to buy lunch elsewhere or bring lunch in and didn't have to rely on the federally subsidized NSLP. In this way, the cafeteria was an intervention in inequality—a means to minimize the field of stigma, address diet-related health disparities, and craft a public space to be shared by students from often dramatically different worlds of opportunity and advantage. This frame of understanding became crystal clear as I listened to her talk about the space of the cafeteria. At one point in our interview, she referred to the cafeteria as "the great equalizer," a statement she had also overheard other administrators use. "Everybody eats side by side," she explained. "You don't think that it's just the poor kids who are eating lunch. Everybody eats lunch here, you know. Right now we're feeding about thirteen hundred reimbursement lunches. We're feeding several hundred kids who just want a piece of pizza." This all took on special significance because in academic spaces in school, segregation abounds. In truth, there was a lot of social segregation in the cafeteria, not just in classrooms, which is a theme I address in the next chapter. Some kids brought lunch from home to stay above the fray, to opt out of the scene altogether. But they did in fact share the space, stand in the same lines, and, more or less, eat the same food.

Brenda's characterization of the cafeteria as "the great equalizer" was more than just empty rhetoric. A moral language of doing right by the students infused Brenda's accounting of her work. For Brenda the idea that the cafeteria could be an equalizing space, like the promise of public education itself, was a means to effect steady, incremental, and lasting change—in other words, to achieve what she regarded as real change in and through one of our most sacred, but also much maligned, public institutions, school.

School Food and Food Justice

The idea of the cafeteria as a vehicle for positive change was a means for Brenda to create value in her work. When I first sat down with Brenda to interview her, she asked me if my project was a "food justice project." Because it didn't, in fact, begin as one, I remarked that I was interested in food justice as part of the larger project. Frankly, I was surprised by her question. I am certain that my own assumptions about school food directors informed my thinking. Brenda challenged many of my early assumptions. Her question signaled a particular conception of her work, its social mission and its moral motive. She understood that health and children's well-being were indelibly linked to hunger, food insecurity, and family resources and that school, as a public institution, could have meaningful impact in addressing public health.[35] Brenda demonstrated a keen appreciation of the way income disparities in families manifest as diet-related health disparities. "When apples are $1.89 a pound and three apples is a pound. What are you going to buy to fill your kids up? Chips or an apple? It's a sad state of affairs." Brenda explained the impact for her school: "When we first started, we were feeding about 65 percent of our reduced-eligible children. We now feed between 85 percent and 90 percent of our reduced-eligible children," thereby maximizing student participation.[36]

The school cafeteria was a space for students to be introduced to new foods and cultivate a taste for healthy foods, which was especially meaningful since so many students were part of groups often referred to as "the new hungry," those whose access to healthy food options are limited even as their access to foods more generally are not. In addition to introducing students to new nutrient-rich foods, the cafeteria offered culturally recognizable foods. Plantains and *yuca* (baked not fried), both staples of a South American diet, were offered as a means to connect with the large and growing immigrant base of students from Central and South America. Traditional southern offerings such as sweet potatoes and collard greens were offered as a kind of comfort food to a large base of African American students, many with deep roots in southern cooking.[37] The effort to provide familiar, ethnic-based foods was a means to reach kids where they are. This strategy of inclusion reminded me of anthropologist Margaret Mead, who in the 1940s served as chairwoman for the Committee on Food Habits for the USDA. Working to preserve ethnic differences in food practice, Mead promoted "food choice" as an alternate to the heavy-handed efforts to promote Americanization through food served in lunchrooms.[38]

Yet Brenda was often seen as a tough nut to crack by some of the food movement actors and concerned parents in the community wanting to launch more progressive food programs, expand healthy, sustainable, locally sourced food options, and expand a school garden program in the school district.[39] And while people working to advance local, sustainable, farm-to-school movement goals often lamented that Brenda could do more, I often felt as though the two camps were not so far apart in their goals. Both cared deeply about health. Both recognized that health disparities were rooted in economic inequalities. Both seized on the school as an institutional setting to address inequalities that shape food access and limit food justice.

Brenda's accounting of her work serves as a reminder that the public provisioning of food in schools is bound to ideas about responsibility of care by American public institutions. It is easy to lose sight of the role public institutions play in the care of our children in the context of increasing privatization of that care and our current cultural preoccupation with personal responsibility, sometimes at the expense of our collective obligations. Perhaps all of this is the case because food's symbolic dimensions are so weighted with meaning about care. Brenda worked hard to bring into being a food-provisioning system that was caring and just, recognizing students and pushing them to be better versions of themselves.

Reforming School Food

While the National School Lunch Program (NSLP), officially adopted in 1946 as a federal mandate, has been a topic of contestation since its beginning, never have American public schools been subject to such intense and widespread scrutiny over matters of food as they are today. As Brenda offered in the characteristic no-nonsense tone I came to appreciate, "The image of school nutrition is poor. Period." And she's right. This chapter has examined public food provisioning at Thurgood High School, a large, racially mixed school where 60 percent of its students are eligible for free or reduced lunch, and where addressing health and hunger are school district priorities. This chapter highlights the compromises and struggles involved in bringing such a system of care into being from the perspective of what it looks like on the ground.

Historian Susan Levine reminds us that struggles over states' rights during the mid-twentieth century were fundamental to political conflicts over school lunch, over what was served, who got to eat, and who ultimately footed the bill. So too do larger political struggles come to bear on the organization of school lunch today. Food and beverage industries have gone to great lengths to maximize youth appeal in both their marketing and their product development, though shaping, often narrowly, the range of possibilities for youth and children.[40] Yet, a careful look at Thurgood reveals that the specific unfoldings of these larger currents are deeply local in character and form.[41] Thus while markets are important institutional players in the crafting of school lunch, making food appealing is bound up with specific social arrangements of cultural milieu as well. At Thurgood, the idea of students as customers was harnessed by the food director to improve the way students, most of whom were low-income and of color, were treated by the food service workers she supervised, to mitigate what sociologist Allison Pugh (2009) has termed "dignity injuries." Brenda's conception of students as customers was a rallying call to extend to these students the dignity and respect people expect to receive in the marketplace.[42] Student choice and a focus on trend profiles resonant with youth tastes were things that Brenda paid attention to as she planned the menus. With the support of her school administration, Brenda went to great lengths to make food appealing to the kids, at the same time that she remained committed to providing healthy food options.[43]

While all food stations were modeled after commercial equivalents, as Brenda told me with notable pride, all the foods are lower in salt, sugar, and fat than their commercial counterparts. An ethic of care guided her efforts to address hunger and health, to value the kids themselves, and to recognize the life circumstances that might prevent them from having sufficient access to healthy food options. At Thurgood, the challenges were many. Not only was the scale of operations substantial but also concern over the stigma of hunger and poverty hung in the background. Brenda was aware that sushi, an offering that would be available only for students paying out of pocket and not those participating in NSLP, serves to reinforce established symbolic divisions between those who have the resources to pay for lunch and those without, who must rely on free- and reduced-lunch subsidies. But the program needed to sell sushi and other food items to generate revenue, even if offering this food meant that only a small portion of the kids could afford to buy it.

Market research has demonstrated that teenagers want more ethnic foods in their school cafeterias.[44] But providing ethnic offerings, for Brenda, was also bound up with ideas about ethnic and racial inclusion. The decision to put *yuca* (baked, not fried), a staple starch of a South American diet, on the menu was made in an effort to improve participation for newly arriving immigrant students from South America. It was harnessed as a means to fortify a sense of belonging.[45]

Well aware of the broader political landscape of food, Brenda sought to have measurable impact where she could. She was pragmatic and expressed criticism of school food policy and practice based on what she called a "food philosophy" rather than on evidence-based research. Her references to science were numerous. Her decision about whether to sell flavored milk, for instance, or how to evaluate the nutritional value of school lunch versus lunches brought from home in her district were rooted firmly in a commitment to empirically grounded evidence as a directive for policy and practice.[46] She also saw herself as pushing the envelope. This year Brenda took french fries off the daily menu. Even though the district had never served *fried* french fries, only baked, she saw her actions as "bold" and "audacious" and expected to be "tarred and feathered." While she thought she was "going to hear it," there was "not one comment," perhaps because she replaced fries with roasted potato with rosemary, a tasty alternative.

The cafeteria and its food offerings were ultimately seen as both a means and an end—that is, a vehicle by which to address and alleviate problems of both resource distribution and recognition. The philosopher Nancy Fraser identifies in her theory of injustice two spheres of changeable action: a symbolic sphere where concerns for recognition and respect play out and the socioeconomic sphere, where problems of misdistribution in resources unfold. The symbolic sphere is centered in struggles for visibility and dignity. These commitments to recognition and redistribution were also expressed by other Thurgood administrators, with consequence for the way youth engaged the cafeteria as a school space. In the next chapter, we return to Thurgood's cafeteria, examining how the space was structured for youth ends, with attention to the spatial arrangements of food and eating and how enduring inequalities among students continued to shape the cafeteria, despite efforts to mitigate their influence.

3

The Cafeteria as Youth Space

Social Bonds and Barriers

On a breezy autumn day in late October, I stand in Thurgood's cafeteria just as the bell rings and a scattering of kids begins the rush in from the four corners of the large room, a few practically sprinting in an effort to beat the long lines. Within minutes, the lunch lines extend out the doors. A girl in the grill line, always the longest, turns to her friend: "Line's not so long." "It ain't?" her friend responds doubtingly. Today, the administration has put up queue poles to direct the kids. Mr. Edwards, one of the vice principals, tells me the poles are intended to impose some order in the hopes of reducing both cutting and food theft.[1] A few kids cut anyway, hopping over the belts, and each time, Mr. Edwards walks over and directs them to the end of the line. One girl tries several times to cut; when it is clear she will not succeed, she whirls around and says, "O-K-a-a-y!" in a small yell. Unphased, he directs her to the end of the line again, and seconds later another girl cuts. A boy in a black pea coat stands just beyond the lunch line with tray in hand. Popping a grape into his mouth, he intones with exasperation in the direction of his friend, "Duuude, hurry up," "Dude, cut!" Three girls, all wearing the hijab and holding hands, move patiently through the international food line. The lines continue to build even as other kids exit, making their way with trays to the tables; many kids nibble on their lunch as they walk. In the cafeteria, food doesn't anchor kids in place in the way it might in a restaurant or at home.

A boy exits with pizza and a cookie on his tray, makes a quick stop at a table where he hands over the cookie, slipping it into a girl's bag, then moves on. This is one of the few instances of food gifting I observe during my time at Thurgood. I walk the room, stopping by a booth occupied by six African American kids: three girls, three boys. The largest of the three boys, wearing an oversized green golf shirt, is singing, rather loudly, an excerpt from Eminem and Rihanna's duet, "Love the Way You Lie." His movements are jocular and halting as he affects a kind of tough swagger. The room is bubbling with chatter, and a piercing pitch from one of the tables echoes through the room, followed by bursts of laughter. Several hundred kids occupy the room, which creates an intense acoustic energy. A group of black girls is gathered together at one of the tall bar tables, eating. One girl is sucking on a green lollipop, one of the few food items I see on this day (or any other day, for that matter) that was not bought from the school cafeteria. Few kids bring lunch from home, and even fewer store-bought or fast-food items can be found here.[2]

At one of the tall bar tables a boy with long braids, wearing a white t-shirt and dark indigo jeans, stands shooting the bull with two other boys as they eat, a burger for one, Chinese chicken and rice for the other. A leggy black girl in jeggings, whom I spot on most days, breezes past the table, and the standing boy calls out with a warm, raspy chuckle, "Still struttin' your stuff." She offers a slight smile but does not slow her pace as she walks with purpose around the tables toward the door, passing another large group of seven huddled in a booth. A girl sits on the lap of a boy who mixes ranch dressing and hot sauce on his plastic tray and then dips his pizza in it, a combination I have seen many times here. A girl approaches him but is quickly rebuffed. "No, I can't talk to you right now. I'm eating," he says gruffly, and she turns and heads toward another table without a word.

Unlike at Washington High School, where the bustle of activity resides largely in the center of the room, at Thurgood, the perimeter—that is, the booths—is, in the words of Erving Goffman, "where action is." Vice Principal Edwards told me that the booths were a huge mistake. Kids climb all over them and each other, and too many kids cram themselves into them. I nod, having witnessed this many times myself. On one occasion, I watched four kids stuffed into one side of a booth, one girl leaning over another, and as they playfully wrestled, she opened her mouth and let her saliva drip into the mouth of the other girl. Without a doubt, the booths can get very rowdy.

Cafeterias as Social Spaces

The above scene captures the deeply social character of high school cafeterias. The high school cafeteria is as much about the social encounter as it is about the food. And while the idea that the cafeteria represents a space removed from the academic life of school is misleading, it is true that this is a space where students exercise significant influence, crafting the space as a youth-centered *social* space. Food, not books, serves to define this school setting. Kids travel from classroom to gym, from art to music, stopping along the way for lunch, a thirty-minute break from an otherwise busy, ordered day. At Thurgood, much as with other schools, the lunchroom is a central gathering place, where kids' movements are managed and monitored, but much less closely than in other school spaces, and where books and more often than not teachers are left behind. In this sense, the cafeteria is both a space of control and a space of freedom, a youth space, but mediated by commitments and obligations derived from an adult world. Despite school administrators' best efforts, the cafeteria is likely to be the least orderly of school spaces.[3]

Students at both Washington and Thurgood enjoyed relative freedom, though there were meaningful differences at each of the schools in this regard. At both schools, I watched kids move in and out of the lunch line, in and out of the lunchroom, without comment or hassle. At Thurgood, which is the focus of this chapter, kids move easily from table to table, and some prolong the social dimensions of school by skipping class and hanging out in the cafeteria instead. Given the large space, it's easy to slip in unnoticed and camp out in one of the crowded booths for several lunch periods. At Washington, on the other hand, where the cafeteria is smaller and the noise more easily contained, the cafeteria figures much less as a social destination; kids tend to remain in their seats for the duration of lunch, and kids are much more likely to do schoolwork.

Historically, cafeterias have been heavily monitored. Many high school cafeterias were sex segregated in the 1950s, a result of increasing anxiety about a perceived collapse of a traditional gender order, according to historians.[4] Even today, many schools impose far greater restrictions on students than what I observed at Washington and Thurgood.[5] While many elementary schools assign children to tables and even seats for lunch, most high school students are free to sit with whomever they please. This is not without its own set of dilemmas since there is no guarantee a student will have someone with whom to eat.[6] More than once, I watched kids eat lunch alone. I remember most vividly an eighth-grade boy from Washington, small for his age, who ate alone most days I observed. He was one of the first to arrive and usually finished before the majority of kids sat down, and thus was left to sit idle, watching and waiting for lunch to end. That he was African American in a sea of mostly white kids made his unhappy fate of a lunch spent alone all the more troubling. Nor is this freedom to choose with whom to sit without broader social implications in racially diverse schools, like Thurgood, where segmented integration—that is, the white kids eating at the "white table," black kids eating at the "black table"—is common, which is a theme explored in this chapter.[7]

At both schools, I often watched as early lunch arrivers stood in waiting with tray or bag in hand to see how other students would be grouped by table before committing themselves to any one table, suggesting a careful social calculation. To get the table wrong is to miss out on the break from the academic routine that the cafeteria signifies. As one Thurgood student bemoaned to her friend as she scanned the room, "There ain't no one in this back-ass lunch!" While food can take a back seat to social priorities, a point sometimes lost in discussions around school food reform, it is also true that food is used to facilitate particular kinds of social ties and thus is used for social ends. Food has expressivity. This is what Roland Barthes referred to as the "grammar of food."[8] The forms of sociability in food spaces, the exchange of food that occurs among peers, reveals a complex geography of friendship networks, peer clashes, disses and slights, associations and disassociations, and the cold refusal of recognition of one teen by another. Recall the boy mentioned earlier who refused to talk with the girl because he was eating. It is in this context that race, gender, disability, and class materialize. The willingness to hand over your free or reduced lunch, which was something I witnessed girls gift to boys at Thurgood, is an action steeped in enduring gendered scripts of feminine sacrifice and servitude, for instance.

This chapter examines the social uses of the cafeteria, the geography of groups, and the symbolic role of food for the cafeteria as a youth cultural space where group boundaries relevant to youth materialize. Attention is paid to the means by which social categories that are central to understanding what anthropologist Jennifer Tilton has called "the divided landscape of childhood" are formed in the interactions that unfold around lunch.[9] Youth's engagement with the space of the cafeteria at Thurgood was visibly structured by a set of relations and ties forged to school, as a public institution that at once sorts by race, gender, and class and at the same time attempts to leverage its resources to intervene in and reshape the reproduction of inequalities arising from them. It is in this sense that racial identification is magnified in part by the strategies used to address inequalities in school. At the same time, the social workings of the cafeteria at Thurgood reflected an effort to craft this as a youth space, separated from the academic spaces of the school to promote greater inclusion of those most at risk of being marginalized.

Thurgood's Lunchroom and the Low-Achievement Label

I observed Thurgood High School in the fall of 2010, the year after their unlucky designation as "a persistently low-achieving school," a government classification created to address chronic academic achievement problems. Such schools were supposed to receive additional resources. In Thurgood's case, two million dollars in federal resources were to be invested to reverse what was seen as a downward trend in several measures of academic achievement. The sweep of changes and their effect on the dynamics of the school cafeteria were profound.

For Thurgood, this designation as persistently low achieving came as a surprise, not because they had not had problems with an achievement gap—every administrator and teacher I spoke with acknowledged that point—but because the narrative they created about themselves was one focused on their academic achievements and the rigor of their AP offerings. Within the first few weeks of my observing lunch, I listened to frequent academic boasts; I learned that they had been placed on the *Washington Post*'s "Challenge Index," which measures the number of Advanced Placement course offerings; that they had once received a Department of Education Excellence Award; and that at one point they held one of the highest numbers of National Merit Scholarship semifinalists.[10]

A more accurate characterization than low achieving, however, is that of a wide achievement *gap*, alternately called an "opportunity gap," which the historical legacy of racial discrimination and enduring problems of poverty and disadvantage help us to understand. The school defines itself as a space of racial integration, yet who excels academically still tends to be predicted by race and class.[11] A small percentage of students, largely white and part of the professional middle class, excels academically. Many in this subset of students go on to elite colleges and universities, leaving behind a much larger base of lower-income students, mostly of color.[12] One research report found that while 55 percent of white girls attending Thurgood reported having an A or A- grade point average, less than 20 percent of black boys or girls reported the same.[13] While the school boasts having one of the highest numbers of AP courses in the state, participation rates in AP courses are overdetermined by race at Thurgood, with 20 percent of black students and 25 percent of Hispanic students participating in AP courses in contrast to 50 percent of Asians and 70 percent of white students.[14] As Jacob, a Thurgood student, explained, other than white kids and a small group of South Asian immigrants, "really no kids of other races [were] in any of my classes because I was in all honors and AP classes."

In this way, race gets mapped onto socioeconomic status with meaningful consequences for the achievement gap they are now working to address, as well as the racial and class maps of the cafeteria. In fact, this point became a matter of concern as the school administration weighed the possibility of extending off-campus privileges to students for lunch. Vice Principal Edwards, the administrator with whom I spoke the most, told me that the school administration was entertaining the idea of trying to make the campus open to some of the kids but admitted they weren't quite sure how to do it. Grade point average (GPA) alone, he explained, could not be the central criterion because then it would look as though the administration was favoring one racial group. It will be "a pretty homogenous mix of kids," he offered. In light of the widely acknowledged achievement gap in test scores and GPA (as much a consequence of class as of racial inequality), the effect would be that many more white than black and brown students would be entitled to off-campus privileges.

Following the designation, the school board acted swiftly to address the achievement gap. Strategies were set in motion: smaller classrooms, more professional development for teachers, more intensive tutoring for students, and the beginning of a weekend annex school for the kids most at risk of dropping out.[15] A new principal came in with a new set of rules: no hats, no cell phones, and no iPods.[16] The rules were seen by staff as largely a symbolic response to disciplinary problems. The school also hired a new dean of students to focus exclusively on student issues and not academic ones.[17] Relationship development, as opposed to punitive measures, has been seen as a cornerstone of the positive change they sought. Under this formula, teachers were to be responsible only for instruction, but the task of maintaining social order in the halls and the cafeteria was to be left to the dean of students.[18]

For schools awarded the distinction "persistently low achieving," the stigma weighs heavily upon them. During my time in the Thurgood cafeteria, I often had the sense that the administrators were in a race against time to correct their image as a low-achieving school, to narrow the achievement/opportunity gap and restore their former public identity as "high achieving." Anybody working in public education today understands that in a context where resources hinge on student achievement, the stakes are high. Should they fail, they risk the loss of federal funds and the prospect of closure, and even risk tipping the scales in favor of greater flight of high-achieving, higher-income kids to private schools or better public schools. As Jacob offered, "If that happens, then that's going to ruin Thurgood, because then all the white kids. . . . Parents who could if they wanted to send their kids to private school will and that'll be the end. After that it'll just be some inner-city school with an abysmal academic record." A declining school often translates into declining fortunes and eclipsing the promise of mobility through education.

Worry over a demographic shift in the student population, often characterized in terms of "white flight," and the low-achievement designation structured the cafeteria meaningfully.[19] I remember early in my observations arriving to the cafeteria and spotting an electronic ticker-tape (much like those used in Wall Street brokerage houses) mounted to the stairwell in the center of the cafeteria that read, "Thurgood, where it's cool to be in school." It reminded me of the branding efforts of New York City public schools to convince kids that eating fruits and vegetables was also cool. Sometimes these efforts to recast schools as cool are half-baked, but when carefully executed can be effective in reshaping definitional boundaries, such that something previously regarded as colossally uncool might be renamed as something else.[20] This was especially important since the changes the school sought depended on student buy-in.

Officially acknowledged as the center of school life, the cafeteria served as a strategic setting toward that end. It was a central point of contact between administrative staff and students. In effect, the cafeteria was a setting where academic considerations could be secondary to nurturing relationships of respect and care, increasingly recognized as central to students' long-term investment and success in school.[21] I witnessed many instances where connections were sought and a gentle arm of authority was demonstrated by administrative faculty.[22] "Ladies and gentlemen, let's go, let's go"; "Let's get to class on time"; "Ladies, lunch is now over"; and "Don't let us see you at another lunch" were declarations I heard at the end of lunch nearly every day I observed, delivered by the calm but firm voice of one the vice principals through his bullhorn.

The tone and type of talk projected an easy, respectful rapport, a feeling of "I'm on your side."[23] One afternoon I watched as the dean of students, "Mr. James," a trim, handsome black man in his late thirties dressed in well-tailored clothes, talked with a black student sitting at a table, her school-issued laptop open. I noted a quiet confidence as he leaned over and told her in an assuring but serious tone that she "needs to step it up." She nodded, slowly peeling her eyes away from her computer to recognize him and his request. A few minutes later, another girl came over to Mr. James saying pleadingly, "Someone stole my friend's lunch number and he can't get food!" Mr. James remained calm but took her seriously. He told her to go get her friend and she dragged over a skinny brown boy with black-rimmed glasses, and Mr. James escorted him to the lunch line. On another occasion, I watched as one of the black male administrators told a transgendered kid sternly but with warmth, "Don't let me catch you with that smoothie outside of here." The kid laughed and continued to drink his smoothie but quickened the pace at which he drank. In another instance, I watched as one male administrator, also black, greeted a male student, "What's up man?" Making eye contact and exhibiting a cool authority, he told the boy, "You need to put your cell away." At another lunch, the same administrator called out to a boy, "Don't make me use your middle name." In another instance, a black male student dressed in jeans and red t-shirt was approached by a white male teacher who extended his arm to shake hands—in a street style that communicated recognition of the student as an equal. The student in turn extended his hand and they began to talk. The teacher, emulating a kind of urban youth-speak, asked, "For real?" and the student responded, "For real." The following example, recorded toward the end of lunch, is especially illustrative. A group of three black girls had been singing to themselves, harmonizing a chorus from a pop song as they moved toward the exit. A few feet from them was one of the administrators, who held in her hand a microphone, which she normally used to direct students back to class in an orderly fashion. But on this occasion, she extended the mic toward the girls, who quickly seized the moment to perform the melody for a much larger crowd than they had anticipated. It was a moment of warm connection shared among them. On more than one occasion, I observed girls cry to male administrators who lent a sympathetic ear. Many sociologists will recognize these interactions as examples of a form of symbolic deference that those with power and authority show toward those without—what Erving Goffman identified as central to the status rituals that govern social action and maintain social order.[24]

These examples were part of the normal round of interactions I observed in the cafeteria. For administrators, the cafeteria was seen as a meaningful space to offer recognition, to counter the symbolic violence community and schools can inflict on its most marginalized. This sort of work, which could appropriately be called "dignity work," whereby recognition is bestowed by those who hold institutional power, teachers and staff, to those without, that is, students, was taken up by nearly all the adults to be found in the cafeteria on any given day and helped to define the cafeteria as a space entirely separate from the other school spaces.[25] These types of dealings also provided counterstrategies to the often punitive and policing tactics that sociologists have documented as central to neoliberal governance and that youth of color face in their schools and communities, serving to criminalize them and narrow and erode future possibilities.[26]

When Things Get Rowdy: Play in Liminal Space

Of course, for students at Thurgood, the cafeteria represents something entirely different. A hotbed of activity and noise, the cafeteria sometimes even gets downright raucous as kids seize the space for play and fun. The lunch line, slow-moving and jam-packed, was a particularly rambunctious zone; voices were loud, with kids screaming to be heard. Students flitted from table to table, sitting, talking, standing around, hugging, jostling, and dancing in place, sometimes eating. In this way, the cafeteria is a liminal sphere—at once a school setting and a setting much more profoundly social in its logic, where opportunities for play abound and boundaries are tested.[27] Food and the body, both social objects, are often used as resources to define youth spaces as liminal. At Thurgood, the body is used in dramatic fashion to lay claim to space, to alter, rearrange, and rework space, and thus to transform its meaning. Cutting in line, ducking under or over the line dividers, walking over booths and cramming into them, climbing over other kids, or "copping a feel" can be seen during any given lunch period and contribute to a sense of controlled chaos, whereby clear patterns of permissible behavior are constantly being negotiated, and the borders and boundaries of personal space and group territories are pushed and prodded. This was central to crafting the cafeteria as a liminal social space apart from school. I observed a fair amount of clowning. In one instance, a table of boys had quickly turned around a chair just as one boy prepared to sit in it, so that the back of the chair rested against the table. This required the boy to spread his legs as though mounting a horse, but because he was wearing such sagging jeans that hung well below his hips, he was unable to do so in order to sit in the chair. This was met with hysterical laughter by the other boys, as well as the boy himself. In another instance, that is perhaps not so funny, three girls were standing in line. One was wearing a very short tunic dress that, unbeknownst to her, was in a flash pulled up by the other two, thereby exposing her underwear. At another lunch that same day, I watched a girl run up behind a boy as she tightly clasped her hands around his long braids, directing him to walk in small circles, which he obliged with a bemused look on his face.

For the most part, the school administration was willing to honor the definition of the space that the students sought to advance: the cafeteria as a liminal youth space. In this space, students had significant latitude in terms of bodily comportment. Students moved freely; efforts to contain and to discipline the adolescent body by adults in school were suspended in the cafeteria. The school administration was deliberate in finding alternative ways to discipline students beyond punitive strategies that have the effect of criminalizing students of color, especially boys.

This was no doubt a reflection of the school's broader strategy to nurture students' attachment to and sense of belonging in school.

Yet this strategy allowed old patterns of gender asymmetry, whereby masculine displays and control of space figured prominently, to creep in. One such example was the routine and ritual enactment of conflict play, a sort of staged, rough, dramatized play that often dissolved into a hug, a handshake, or a laugh, but sometimes intensified. This rough play usually took the form of boy on boy, but also boy on girl. In conflict play, dramatized violence is expressed as bodies come into close contact and the definition of what precisely is going on is precarious; dramatizations or stagings that begin as play can morph into genuine expressions of conflict, though this happened only occasionally. During the several months I observed lunch, I witnessed countless fakeouts—punches, slaps, fingers molded as guns pretending to shoot—that threatened violence that never materialized. In one instance, I watched as two boys, one with long dreads, stood together by the food lines, which is a high-visibility area since a majority of students pass through the lunch lines. The skinny boy kept some distance, circling a much bigger boy, moving in and out as he declared, "Take that, bitch," as the bigger boy pretended to absorb a punch. After a few minutes, the encounter transformed as the larger boy grew tired of the game and brought it to a swift close with his sobering expression. In another case, I watched a boy grab a banana from a girl's lunch tray and hold it sideways like a gun, gangster style, to another girl's head. She laughed at this, though it was not clear whether her laugh was genuine. He did it a second time before returning her banana to her, the group's chatter continuing unabated. In another instance a boy pretended to a stab a girl in the neck with a pen.

Because boundaries around bodies are ever shifting and only loosely defined, they are often easily crossed; "play claims" are cast in doubt.[28] I watched boys cop a feel on a girl's behind more than once, with the boy usually feigning innocence, thereby maintaining the claim of play. Yet I also saw girls challenge the play claim. One girl, with a deep scowl on her face, took a swing at a boy, bringing the exchange to an end. On another day toward the end of one lunch, I watched as an exchange between a boy and a girl unfolded as students quickly filed out of the lunchroom. He had cornered her around a table. She went left, he went right, she went right, he went left. This continued for a few minutes, and

I watched as she at first attempted a giggle, smiling politely in an effort to diffuse the situation without making a fuss. But he was unrelenting, smiling as he continued to close off her escape routes. Looking increasingly distressed, her smile now gone, she finally let out a meek, "Stop." With a broad, devilish smile, he persisted for a minute more, bringing the "play" to a close with laughter, presumably thinking all of this was aboveboard. She turned, her face crinkling in a mix of stress and relief, grabbed her bag, and fled the room. Here the exchange moved in a more alarming direction, drifting toward intimidation, while still masked as play. In instances like these, boys impose their bodies on others and in doing so, claim control over large portions of the space and those within it. These assertions of masculine control and physical dominance reflect, and at the same time reinscribe, troubling gender schemes that leave unchecked male claims of entitlement to and control over girls' bodies.

It is difficult to determine whether these actions are expressions of gendered violence exclusively or reflect the working out through play of narratives about routine violence in these students' lives and communities more generally.[29] As Jody Miller in her book *Getting Played* argues, violence is a routine aspect of daily community life in disadvantaged communities. Girls living in communities marked by significant disadvantage are at a higher risk of sexual harassment and sexual assault and are also more likely to witness violence between intimate partners in public. Schools are community institutions and thus, as Miller suggests, "[T]here is good reason to suspect that sexual harassment and its consequences may be especially acute in the school setting." Miller characterizes gender violence as "an everyday feature of the cultural milieu of school" that is "highly public in nature" and routinely "occurred in the presence of other students."[30] While boys tend to interpret this as "harmless play," girls describe these actions as "troubling," "offensive," and "disrespectful."

Much of this passes unnoticed by the administration, however. I observed only two occasions when administrators actively intervened in this "conflict play" during the several months I spent observing in the cafeteria. I am reluctant to suggest that the lack of responsiveness by school staff was due to their being unconcerned. In the two cases where intervention occurred, it was swift and intended to protect the student victimized. Perhaps a better explanation can be found in what the school hoped to achieve through the cafeteria. In many ways, the administration honored young people's effort to craft this space as one of their own, as a liminal youth space, acknowledging it as something other than school, and thus giving students a wide berth in which to anchor themselves to school. Recall the findings from the student focus groups organized by Brenda and discussed in the last chapter. The kids wanted the cafeteria to not feel like school. Honoring this request, the school administration sought alternative ways beyond punitive control to manage students in school, since punitive strategies often have the effect of criminalizing students of color, especially boys, and thus undermining their sense of attachment to school.[31]

But in doing so, they were unable to see the gendered dimension of rough play, allowing what might be seen as smaller infractions to pass without discipline in order to avoid punitive control and remain focused on forging meaningful relationships with students who face the greatest roadblocks to mobility. The effect, however, is to construct the cafeteria as a deeply gendered space where girls' movements are constrained and the freedom to fully seize the cafeteria as a social space is thwarted. The lack of intervention, whether intentional or not, normalized the behavior of those boys who sought to exercise their muscle over girls and other boys, leaving them to fend for themselves.

Why Are the White Kids Eating Together?

Despite these gendered relations, however, time spent in the cafeteria was often the highlight of the students' day; many returned more than they were supposed to, some cutting class to do so. Yet this characterization could mask the indifference to the scene demonstrated by other groups of students. In truth, deep polarization was visible in the cafeteria, manifest in who bought or brought lunch, where they sat, and with whom they ate. For example, youth with cognitive disabilities were largely excluded from the social scene, while youth with physical disabilities were integrated much more fully. While students with more severe cognitive disabilities were required by administrators to eat lunch in their classroom because the scene was recognized as too precarious for them, other students with cognitive impairments were permitted to eat in the cafeteria but were largely consigned to their own tables and were excluded from many of the social dimensions of play. The extent to which students seized the cafeteria as a social space also reflected firmly etched ethno-racial lines that were often difficult to disentangle from the machinations of gender and class.

In the title of her book, psychologist Beverly Tatum asks *Why Are All the Black Kids Sitting Together in the Cafeteria?* while recognizing that white kids are also inclined to group themselves by race. This is a question I also came to ask after I began observing at Thurgood. On the surface, Thurgood is a racially diverse school. And while the Thurgood cafeteria was optimistically regarded as the "great equalizer" by Brenda, the food director, it was also a space of meaningful social divisions.[32] In this way, the same racial and class inequalities responsible for the achievement/opportunity gap discussed earlier also organized the racial maps of students in Thurgood's cafeteria.[33]

Though there certainly were plenty of racially mixed tables that dotted the room (an important point not to be lost), more common were distinct ethno-racial clusters of kids. Scholars of race refer to this phenomenon as segmented integration, whereby different racial groups may occupy the same institutional setting, but often remain separated on some fundamental level. Immigrant kids from South America usually sat together in the corner of the large room, claiming about five tables among themselves. They were easily identified by their distinct Central American style: slicked hair, faded jeans, leather jackets, and studded belts for boys; cascading hair, fitted jeans and tops, and dark eyeliner for girls. Their cultural style, combined with their fluent Spanish, announced their status as immigrants.[34]

Black kids, who represented the largest ethno-racial group, mostly claimed the booths on both sides of the room, though they were also scattered in the more racially integrated zones around the tall-bar tables.[35] Three large tables in the center of the room were consistently claimed by a group of white kids, a group whose cultural style would probably be recognized as "modern preppy," epitomized in the popular and pricey clothing brands they wore: Hollister, Gap, and Abercrombie and Fitch. These racial maps, though often fluid, patterned these different groups' relationships to this setting.

As a psychologist, Tatum identified the increasing salience of race to the identity projects of youth at this specific developmental stage as most relevant to understanding this phenomenon.[36] Sociologists have tackled this same question, identifying a multitude of factors in play—institutional mechanisms of academic tracking, interpersonal dimensions of peer groups, and the force of identity dynamics—for an explanation of how these divisions come into being. Julie Bettie's ethnographic study of white and Mexican American girls coming of age in California's Central Valley provides a rich example of the performative dimensions of youth identities as they take shape within different school settings. Bettie's particular focus is the way class identity is formed as it intersects with gender, sexuality, color, and ethnicity for these two groups as they negotiate classroom dynamics, the meaning of academic achievement, and the symbolic boundaries that form distinct peer networks. Girls whose parents worked as migrant workers rarely formed friendships with the girls whose parents were members of the professional classes. These two groups rarely found themselves in the same classrooms and came to embrace different styles of dress and demeanor in school. Thus, self-identification with particular cultural styles (e.g., hair, make-up, clothes, cars) and conceptions of themselves as students became grounds for the performance of class and racial-ethnic identities by the two groups of girls and helped to explain the racial segmentation in school. Bettie demonstrates the complexity of identity performances as these girls position themselves within their school's academic hierarchy and in so doing, reveals how intimately connected the construction of youth's social identities in school is to the reproduction of social inequalities in school.

Since academic spaces are stratified by race and class, as years of educational research have documented, it stands to reason that we can also expect a stratified arrangement in other school settings, such as the cafeteria. What's more, given that friendship groups are formed with classmates, a majority of school-aged kids will form friendships with kids in the same academic track. If a school has academic tracks sorted by race and class, as Thurgood does, then we can also expect other school spaces to be sorted by the same logic, as Bettie also found.[37] Indeed, spatial arrangements contribute to racial-identity salience. It is in this context that the interactional and cognitive processes through which symbolic distinctions, often called "boundary work," create what sociologist Eviatar Zerubavel refers to as "traditional islands of group identity."[38] Spatial boundaries, stylistics boundaries, and interactional boundaries were easy to see at Thurgood.

At Thurgood, the advanced academic tracks were dominated by white kids. Yet, the cafeteria space was not. Instead, the white kids, many part of the upper-middle class, in the advanced academic tracks congregated in the very middle of the room, an island of relative quiet surrounded by a sea of excitement. Thus, while these kids laid claim to academic spaces, they failed to engage the space of the cafeteria. Residing in the center of the room, away from where the action unfolded, these students were able to successfully avoid contact with other students and opt out of the scene altogether. They were never stragglers, but departed lunch as soon as it drew to a close. "We are out of here," I overheard one of the boys utter at the end of lunch. In time I began to think his words capture a view that was not his alone.

I remember that when I first began observing, I was often overwhelmed by the sense of pandemonium. I had difficulty seeing the relative inaction of this group of students, huddled together at a small collection of tables in the middle of the room. I had become aware that the borders of the room where the booths were was the center of activity. I had already had an earful from the administrators: the booths were a big headache; they seemed to invite chaos.[39]

The center of the room stood in sharp contrast. Kids sat quietly talking, often working on homework, indifferent to the activity unfolding around them. This was most apparent one day when a fight broke out between two girls near the lunch line. Kids seated in booths on both sides of the room stormed the corner where the fight was unfolding, in a fast and furious rush to witness the action. The room's volume rose mercurially, except in the center of the room, where the two tables of almost entirely white kids, guys and girls together, remained unmoved by the unfolding drama. Talking quietly among themselves, they did not turn a single head. Instead, they continued to work on their homework.

Watching day after day, I couldn't help but see their ambivalence as a dramatization. With calculus books as props, they symbolically privileged academics over the social, and in doing so, invoked a posture of indifference to the scene. Refusing to honor the definition of the situation as given by other students enabled them to remain effectively above the fray and in some sense is reflective of a broader retreat by the white upper-middle class from public institutions more generally.[40]

This, I would like to suggest, stems from an ambivalence among high-achieving, white, middle-class kids, nicely captured in Jacob's assessment of the order of things:

> I definitely feel that I would have gotten more attention from the administration had I gone elsewhere. It felt to me like the administration just ignored the white kids for the most part and focused on I guess the underprivileged kids, especially, um, you know, a white kid in all honors and AP classes, he's fine, he doesn't really need, you know, assistance. Let's work on, you know, the 60 percent of kids who can barely pass SOLs [standards of learning] standardized tests.[41]

Given that these students were unable to access the privileges of the sustained educational attention they might enjoy at a private school, and perhaps were not fully aware of their teachers' attention and investment, one can see how a sense of ambivalence toward school as a public institution might take root.[42] This is probably exacerbated by the fact that these students, outside academic spaces, garner less visibility in the school than they might if they were students at more racially homogenous schools, for instance. At racially mixed schools, the social structure among students tends to be more horizontal than vertical, with dispersed lattice-like networks instead of hierarchical ones.[43] Other sociologists have observed that the geographically bounded experiences of white, middle-class students in racially and economically diverse schools results in relatively homogenous social networks among them, thereby undermining the democratic function of inclusive and integrated public schools.[44]

In some ways, these white students are very much like the upper-middle-class jocks in Penelope Eckert's classic book *Jocks and Burnouts,* which compared the way class shaped students' orientations toward school. She found that upper- and middle-class kids were astute in performing the public role of student, deferential to prevailing definitions of school, especially in comparison with the working-class kids who publicly rejected school authority. Joe Foley similarly found in a Texas public school with a predominantly Mexican American student body that the upwardly mobile Mexican American students largely succeeded in school because they knew how to project a performance of conforming students, invested in school while in the presence of adult authority, even if in their private peer interactions, they were more critical of school.

These Thurgood students differentiated themselves in their dress and demeanor, easily embodying an image of a clean-cut, academically oriented student. In addition to seizing the lunchroom space as a place to do homework, thereby maintaining a posture of academic commitment even in nonacademic space, the majority brought lunch from home. Bringing lunch from home enabled students to opt out of the broader lunch scene, an act that also visibly demonstrated their independence from a subsidized lunch system.[45]

Of course, the reasons why kids bring lunch from home are many: allergies, dislike of food offerings, worry of being assigned stigma, concern for calories, and/or cost. And the meaning of bringing lunch from home is context driven. It can serve to communicate to others that you do not rely on free or subsidized lunch, which often carries a poverty stigma. Marcus Weaver-Hightower, in his research on school lunch in the poor townships of Pretoria, South Africa, found that the ability to bring lunch from home signaled status for kids. Since free lunch is offered to all children irrespective of income in South Africa and in the poor townships carries little to no stigma or shame, being able to bring lunch from home is a distinct mark of pride.[46]

At Thurgood, whether the effect was intended or not, bringing lunch from home was a way to hover above the fray, since it enabled students to avoid the uproarious commotion of the lunch lines and avoid contact with those who stood in them, that is, lower-income kids, many of them immigrants and of color.[47] This seemed particularly salient for white girls, who rarely if ever bought lunch, and hints at how the dynamics of a race and gender order belonging to another period of history can endure over time and meaningfully influence the lives of contemporary youth.

Day after day, I watched the same group of white girls, easily identified by their long, straight hair and similar style of dress, move quietly and deliberately with brown lunch bags in hand through the crowded clusters of kids arriving to lunch and into their seats, where they remained for the entire lunch period. While one might be quick to assume that a lunch brought from home for a group of white girls who are thin and fit is an effort to avoid calories associated with school lunch and is thus explained by a feminine preoccupation with body consciousness, given the ample healthy lunch offerings available for purchase at school and the standard sandwich, apple, and chips most often brought from home, I find this explanation wanting. While no doubt relevant in some cases, such an explanation fails to account for the broader sets of social meanings in play in Thurgood's cafeteria. Instead, gender, class, and race converge in ways that patterns youth's different relationship to each other, shared public institutions like school, and the social spaces and social objects therein.

Sociologists of youth have consistently found that in racially diverse schools much like Thurgood, racial categories and boundaries are central to youth identity processes. For Thurgood students, race was salient in patterning the scene and the way they occupied it, yet it is the case that students often have limited contact with each other across racial groups. Jacob, in the interview quoted above, described how unaware he was of the school worlds many African American and Latino students occupied until he decided to take a summer class in the trades for "easy credit" so he could focus on his advanced placement classes during the school year. This experience provided one of the first occasions for him to be in class with majority African American and Latino students and to forge friendships with them. It was an eye opener, he said, and the effect on him was not unlike what Pam Perry in *Shades of White* found in examining the development of racial consciousness and racial self-concept among white students. She compared white youth identity formation at two different schools: one a racially mixed, minority-white urban high school, similar to Thurgood, and the other, a predominantly white, suburban high school. She found that racial composition, racial association, and physical proximities played a salient role in the formation of a racial self-concept for white students as they navigated the changing landscape of increasing racial diversity in schools. The white kids in Perry's study who attended the racially mixed, minority-white school were much more likely to see being white as a distinct cultural identity, having a distinct cultural style with differing tastes in music and clothing, than the white kids at the nearly all-white school did, and thus were much more likely to see themselves as a distinct group separate from other racial groups. The racial maps easily observable at Thurgood similarly suggest the salience of race in patterning youth cultural style, students' relationships to school, and their friendship groups as they unfold in the cafeteria.

Dilemmas of Public Space: School Lunchrooms, Racial Inclusion, and Unequal Schooling

The last chapter identified market influences on school food, Brenda's struggles to increase school food appeal for kids in order to grow student participation, and the commitment to care that inspired her work. Her efforts served both practical and symbolic ends—keeping the cafeteria afloat; forestalling the possibility that the cafeteria would revert to being a place for poor and near-poor kids alone and instead maintaining its function as a central gathering place for all; and communicating the respect the school had for its students.[48] I often felt as though the school was running a campaign to increase the value students assigned to school and to refocus energy toward those most at risk of being left behind, passed over, pushed through, or pushed out. The cafeteria figured significantly in this project, providing a setting for adults to engage with kids outside the confines of an academic sphere where different forms of evaluation were in play.

Yet for all intents and purposes, the cafeteria was mostly regarded, with some exception, as a space of play, separated out from the academic spaces that defined school and some young people's ambivalence toward it. In this sense, Thurgood had successfully honored students' request that the cafeteria not feel like school. Yet recall also the small group of white, middle-class students, who each day quietly claimed their place at the two large tables in the center of the room, far away from the playful, noisy booths. They almost never bought lunch, thereby avoiding the densely packed lunch lines. Their actions spoke loudly, even if they did not, and expressed their collective disinvestment and disinterest in the cafeteria space as social space, a setting that provides one of the few opportunities in school for interaction across race lines for many students. In this sense, the structuring of the space to strengthen ties and investment to school through the cafeteria for some students may serve to exacerbate the symbolic boundaries between students. The issue of who bought lunch or brought lunch also served to highlight these boundaries. This, in tandem with the institutional mechanisms of sorting students into different academic tracks, means that many students leave Thurgood having experienced entirely different schools. In this way, racial integration celebrated at diverse schools like Thurgood still must find better ways to realize public education's potential promise of achieving greater equality.

4

Eat What's Good for You

Class and the Cult of Health

It is late morning on a warm June day in 2010 as Washington High School students start to trickle into the lunchroom—maybe sixty kids as opposed to the several hundred at Thurgood— quietly filtering into two lines that stretch out the double doors that connect the cafeteria to the kitchen, where two steam tables are loaded with pulled pork and what look like cheese steak sandwiches. There are other offerings— applesauce, strawberry sauce, canned peaches at the salad bar, which has tuna salad, lettuce, cucumbers, tomatoes, kidney beans, and chickpeas, an assortment of dressings in small packets, and pita bread slices. Kids can get sandwiches—turkey and cheese or tuna salad. There is fat-free milk and chocolate milk, Switch, a 100 percent fruit juice sparkling soda. On this particular day, there is no ice cream, pizza, french fries, or cookies—the standard fare at a large number of American public schools. Many students in line are with cell phone in hand, one boy holds a lacrosse stick, and another carries a saxophone case. A boy chimes from the back of the line, "Open the flood gates." "Oh man, I'm not eating," I hear another boy lament as he inspects the offerings, picks up a milk, and heads past the salad bar to the cashier. A few minutes later I overhear a boy exclaim, "Yes! This is the best lunch they have." Though he has brought lunch from home, in his excitement, he blurts, "I may not be able to pass it up." He doesn't. Joe, the security guard, in his baritone voice, calls from across the room, "Two lines," a reminder to maintain a semblance of order. Kids mostly fall into easy formation.

Several students, upon entering the room, head directly toward a table, bypassing the lunch line altogether. Within minutes brown paper bags and fabric lunch bags, signaling a lunch brought from home, litter many tables. One girl, slender, with long blonde hair pulled into a ponytail and dressed in khaki shorts and sandals, plops her floral Vera

Bradley lunch tote on a table top before heading over toward the lunch line.[1] Four other girls sit there already, chatting and giggling as they eat their lunch. Two of the girls have the pulled pork sandwich and a bottle of water, one has a low-fat organic yogurt, and two have milk. I scan the room, spotting two cans of soda, one Coke and one Pepsi, and an iced tea bottle—all purchased outside school, since these cannot be purchased in school, except in the teachers' lounge. Most kids here are drinking bottled water, with a smaller number drinking milk. I see a boy with a bag of Cheetos brought in from the outside, and another boy sits with a bag of potato chips. At many of the tables I see small baggies of carrots and grapes, several sandwiches, and apples, indicating lunch brought from home.

Within the first few minutes of lunch, kids have already gathered into groups of varying size, occupying twelve of the twenty or so tables. As with the other lunch periods, the tables in the center of the room are the most crowded. One table, meant to accommodate eight students, holds about twelve, a mix of boys and girls jammed in with chairs cockeyed, since all cannot fit comfortably around the table. Joe tells me with the assurance of someone who has the lay of the land, "Those are my juniors," as he nods in the direction of the table. As I continue to scan the room, I spot a tall, slender girl with long blonde hair in shorts and a sweatshirt, standing with tray in hand beside a boy, also slender and blonde. They each search the room, conferring quietly. He suggests going outside, but she replies that she is not sure they are allowed. Underclassmen are not allowed to leave the room during lunch, though I never once saw that rule enforced. Later, I see her outside eating her lunch.

The room is abuzz with talk, but a quiet type of talk. Out of the corner of my eye, I spot a group of girls at one of the tables toward the center of the room sharing a microwave popcorn bag as they sit chatting. At the table beside them a boy reaches out his hand, and a boy with a small bag of Kellogg's fruity snacks (an item that can be purchased in the school's vending machines) hands him three pieces in exchange for an apple slice, which he promptly hands over. A few kids are playing cards, a few play games on their phones, and a few sit listening to music. Suddenly a chair drops to the floor—the only incident of noise during the entire lunch beyond the hum of chatter. I watch as a boy with sandy brown hair, a bit awkward in his demeanor, who began his lunch at one table alone, hesitantly gets up and moves to another table. He sits on the edge of his chair, barely a part of the table he is attempting to join, his tray balanced carefully on one knee. He makes a few remarks to the boys closest to him at the table; the three girls at the table completely ignore him. At another table sit four boys. One pulls a Hungry-Man meal box from inside his backpack, his smile widening as he reveals the package to his friends. This is a lunch that deserves notice. He sits for a moment intently reading the print on the box as the other boys at the table provide comment, joking to themselves. His is a rather strange lunch by normal lunch standards, a point of which he seems happily aware. One of the boys at the table chews on a plastic fork. Before lunch's end, it is totally mangled.

There are no seniors here today, Joe, a regular fixture in the lunchroom and one of my primary informants at Washington, tells me. "Never is." Even on rainy days, they stay away, lining up in the senior hallway. Lunch spent in the cafeteria for a senior, soon to be graduating, represents a fate only slightly better than detention, I guess. Unlike Thurgood, Washington is an open campus, though privileges to leave campus during school hours are selectively granted—awarded for seniors as long as they maintain an adequate GPA and have logged a sufficient number of community service hours.[2] Most students at Washington I spoke to agreed that the bar had been set pretty low. Unlike at Thurgood, where there is steady movement as kids hop from table to table, at Washington kids tend to remain seated.[3] This has the effect of crafting a series of micro-scenes contained at individual tables, rather than a torrent of activity, as with Thurgood. Most days I arrived to a cafeteria marked not by the boisterous sounds of cacophony but by a quiet hum.

The unfolding dramas of cafeteria life at Thurgood and Washington were remarkably different in both scale and scope, as was most evident even at the onset of my research. Washington High School, less than ten miles from Thurgood, is much smaller, with just under eight hundred students, and is much less diverse in terms of both income and traditional measures of diversity—race and ethnicity. Over 70 percent of Washington students are white (non-Hispanic), with 11.6 percent Asian or Pacific Islander, 9 percent Hispanic, and 6.2 percent African American.[4] The scale of operations, given the schools' size, differs significantly. Resource rich, Washington is nationally recognized as an academically high-achieving school, having been ranked by *Newsweek* for years because of the high percentage of students who enroll in advanced placement courses. (Several years ago the entire eighth grade moved over to the high school because of the high number of eighth graders needing advanced math instruction.)

My first few visits to Washington were pretty unremarkable.[5] I observed Washington the spring prior to observing Thurgood. In fact, it was Dan, the food director at Washington, who encouraged me to contact Brenda, Thurgood's food director. He thought Thurgood would be interesting for me to observe because the cafeteria was so large, in comparison to Washington, and looked so much like a food court at a shopping mall. In contrast, Washington's cafeteria looks like a school cafeteria, characteristic in its tables and chairs, two vending machines, large trash cans on wheels, and two single lunch lines. The most distinguishing feature of the lunch room is the fifty-plus national flags that hang from the ceiling in a single row from one end of the room to the other and that represent, as the principal explained, students who have attended Washington and thus reflect the school's pride in and commitment to international diversity, despite the relative homogeneity of the student body.

This chapter examines what food represents in this school and the broader community that it helps to anchor, capturing the complex interplay among commercial food markets, public institutions, and private and personal interests. Three types of food can be found on any given day in Washington's lunchroom: home food, school food, and market-based commercial food.[6] Each serves different ends within a matrix of social meaning that binds youth to each other, youth to school, and the school to the community. Washington had undergone significant change in the last several years in terms of what was on the lunch menu, converting what had been the typical "carnival fare" found in most public schools, to borrow from Janet Poppendieck, into an expanding array of healthy food offerings. The transformation in school food arose from increasing parental pressure to replace "unhealthy" foods and to close the distance between the types of food kids eat in and outside of school. At Thurgood, school food was largely treated as a public good to address health and hunger, conceived as a means to correct the deficiencies of community and home. In contrast, school food at Washington was not a corrective to the limits of community and home, but transformed to be more like the food eaten at home, and was used to signal distinction by the school itself. This, I argue expresses the broader class commitment of the community to promote a type of "responsible consumption" of the professional middle class, "distinguished in part by its interest in health, fitness and food," and is emblematic of the way the professional middle class engages with public institutions more generally.[7] Focusing on the food director's effort to transform school lunch and respond to parental demand to do so, I explore a central tension between the prevailing democratic sensibility that public institutions such as schools should serve all equally and advance broader public interests, and the pull of professional middle-class parenting sensibilities to leverage and consolidate public and private resources to give their children the best possible futures, thereby placing pressure on public institutions to bend to their will and adapt to their needs in the process.

The transformations I detail here point to the ambivalent relationship of the professional middle class to public institutions in a period of time linked to neoliberal agendas that privilege the private as superior to the public and advance market-driven solutions to matters once seen as the exclusive domain of public institutions. The first portion of the chapter sketches the changing set of arrangements in food consumption toward a focus on health that Dan, the food director, labored to bring into being and the role of parental pressure in driving such change. The second portion of the chapter shifts attention toward youth, highlighting the way class dispositions shape what kids consume and how they consume and examining how this same ambivalence finds expression in the types of play students engage in this space.

Class, School Food Reform, and the Cult of Health

At the time of my observation at Washington, the district food director, Dan, was in his third year. Dan, a middle-aged black man, had a daughter in high school, though in another school district with more affordable housing for middle-income folks like himself. As part of a new pledge by the school district, Dan had been hired to transform the lunchroom menu—specifically, to expand the base of healthy offerings. Dan came to the job with a lifetime spent in food service, but none in schools. In this sense he was an outsider, new to the politics of who cashes in on soda machines, the USDA commodities surplus program, the "heat and serve" model of food delivery in lunchrooms, debates over the provision of "offer vs. serve," or the challenges of working with a largely deskilled, low-paid occupational group who are often non-English speakers—all of which issues characterize the current constraints of food provisioning of public schools and the National School Lunch Program.[8] At our first meeting, Dan characterized the food served before his arrival as "kids' food: chicken nuggets, pizza, spaghetti, things like that." Dan detailed some of the positive food changes he had been able to accomplish, in particular introducing a popular salad bar. "We do roasted eggplant with alfalfa sprouts with cheese," he told me, proudly adding, "Vegetarians love it."[9]

"I'm working against changing my employees' attitudes about doing something that is just reheating food," Dan explained.[10] Since arriving, Dan had been successful in the retraining of his staff to move away from a "heat and serve" model toward mixed-scratch cooking.[11] His staff now made a low-fat chicken pot pie and cheese quesadillas from scratch, and in this sense the changes expressed many of the culinary virtues of a food culture often associated with the cosmopolitan upper-middle class: hand crafted, simple yet distinctive, improved quality, with a range of ethnic food options.[12]

Some of Dan's changes took both his staff and students by surprise. Ice cream and french fries, which had been previously available for purchase every day, were now only available once a week. Like Brenda, Dan grew to appreciate that slow and steady movement toward progressive change could be lasting. "Evolution, not revolution," he often opined. "You have to really try to balance it. In the beginning I made too much drastic change." The kids rebelled. But after a few fumbles, he turned to the students. "What I found is most kids don't know what they want, they can say that the food sucks or the food's good. 'Well what would you like to eat?' They don't know," Dan explained. "That's because you don't give them the option."

For Dan, the narrow range of options was a consequence of the food industries' constant fleecing of meager school lunchroom budgets, a fair amount of deception on their part in terms of promises on both price and portion size.[13] This, combined with budget shortfalls, often left him up against a wall. Budget constraints were felt daily and were unlikely to change any time soon. He struggled to overcome the limits of school purchasing power by joining a co-op and was looking to incorporate a gourmet food class with his food program. To better circumnavigate the endless budget woes of a food director, he sought creative partnerships with a paraprofessional cooking school and held taste-test competitions with students voting for what they liked most, which the kids enjoyed. The students from the cooking school were tasked to "think of dishes that will fit into my budget." His efforts were not in vain and were featured in a national food service trade magazine. Several times he remarked to me that outsiders had said that if he were in a poor school district, he wouldn't be able to make the changes he had made. But he didn't buy this line of reasoning. His response was that the school district down the road had "the same amount of money and they still give their kids pizza and french fries."

Like nearly all the young people I interviewed, Dan's point of reference against which all cafeteria food was judged was the almighty restaurant, a cultural institution belonging to the private realm of leisure and pleasurable consumption. "I would like to do restaurant-quality food but in my budget . . . eventually," he confided. Dan largely followed a business model, championing growth and expansion, with the aim to maximize visibility and reach.[14] Dan sought to create various community and local business partnerships to minimize budget shortfalls.

Dan was also beholden to the so-called competitive foods, like Pop-Tarts and an assortment of chips, reliant on them to draw students in so as to avoid budget deficits. But Dan was also well aware that competitive food belonging to commercial markets threatened to undermine the sustainability of the National School Lunch Program, an emblem of the democratic access that public school represents.[15] As Dan reported one afternoon, "I know the research: only 20 percent of kids will select the healthy food when presented with the other stuff." The easy access to commercial food outlets for students at Washington because of proximity and the relatively free movement between school and commercial sphere resulting from its open campus policy, combined with the substantial disposable income for a large number of students, presented a distinct problem for Dan as he worked to introduce healthier options in school that met both parental and student approval.

Like Brenda, Dan turned to the private market sphere for answers. He followed market trends and introduced foods with market resonance in innovative ways to gain greater student participation and thus stay financially afloat. Chinese chicken, vegetables, and rice, for example, was served in a Chinese take-out box. Dan understood that the way food was packaged mattered to its appeal, especially for a group of youth who are already active and discriminating consumers. More than anything, the kids seemed to appreciate the box; the food was secondary. In one instance, I observed a girl standing in line who decided against the chicken and rice once she realized they had run out of the Chinese take-out boxes. The challenges for Dan are quite different from Brenda's, however. First, the vast majority of students really do have the option to eat elsewhere since so few are free- or reduced-lunch-eligible and Washington has an open campus, allowing students to eat lunch at any of the many lunch places within a close walk of school. Seniors are largely absent altogether since they are permitted to leave campus. A large number of kids, unlike at Thurgood, bring lunch from home. This was further compounded by the fact that kids seized the cafeteria as a space for socializing; food was secondary. Taken together, these obstacles were ever present as he worked to make the food, especially food that is part of the National School Lunch Program, appealing while also satisfy a healthy-food mandate from parents.

Hypervigilant Parents

A significant part of Dan's work was dealing with the parents, a subject he frequently talked about in a way Brenda simply did not.[16] Life at Washington and indeed the community at large reflects a distinct cultural style and ethos of parental engagement that sociologists largely associate with the affluent and educated.[17] The tree-lined streets and large Craftsman homes that surround Washington are largely populated by those belonging to the professional upper-middle class. Median annual household income is over $100,000, and median home price in 2011 was $630,000.[18] Of course, the high-priced property values are tied in part to the distinctiveness of the high school, secured by the sustained involvement of parents with considerable professional power to exert influence over school policy.[19]

Dan told me about how the parents had led a successful campaign to have plastic trays replaced by corrugated compostable paper trays, despite the significant monthly increase in overhead cost (a sixteen-hundred-dollar difference monthly), for example.[20] One of the first changes Dan made was the items sold in the two vending machines in the cafeteria. He admitted that this action was an eye opener: "I put in my healthy vending machine and parents called me and e-mailed me about it. The kids told me you had new vending machines and the food in it was really healthy and they thought it was cool." This level of response and feedback from parents came as a surprise, as did the fact that this registered as a noteworthy event for parent-child conversation. "I wouldn't go home and talk about food. The vending machine . . . it wouldn't be a conversation piece for me." Quickly, Dan learned to expect regular parental comment.[21] He recalls, "The first time I introduced my frozen drink, I got a lot of e-mails. In this area there are a lot of prominent parents, people who write for *USA Today*. I have to be very careful when I respond before I end up in some publication blasted across the front page!" Dan learned he must tread lightly, must prepare for comment, and had to do his homework well in advance. Gradually he came to conceive of his role as that of an information broker. "Usually when I respond, I'm already right, I have no fear." "I had a parent write me and say, 'Why am I selling Slurpies masquerading as smoothies?'" Dan e-mailed back with the product's nutritional information, noting that it had less sugar than a regular can of juice. Feeling righteous, Dan confided, "They never responded back."

After three years, Dan had learned to be preemptive, anticipating how parents might react to changes being made and maintaining productive ties with a well-organized and active PTA, whose reach in school was significant. "We have healthy muffins now. I introduced it to the two elementary schools, at the PTA meeting before I did it. I told them I was bringing out squash muffins and spinach and yam muffins." Not surprisingly, this was met with significant parental support, though parents did attempt to negotiate how the muffins were described to students. "I encourage everybody to e-mail me. . . . I had one parent who called me and said, 'I don't think the high school should have any sugar whatsoever, they get enough junk food.' I said, 'Unfortunately you're the only one who feels that way.'" Shaking his head with incredulity, he added,

"You cannot eliminate sugar from other kids' diets." Other parents wanted to eliminate sodium, sugar, and fat, but he was a pragmatist. He already had to compete against student clubs, which regularly sell cans of Coke and Krispy Kreme doughnuts, coveted food items among youth, especially in school, for fundraising during school hours.

Dan was talking, though indirectly, about a particular parental orientation to school, sometimes called "intensive parenting," well documented by sociologists and characterized by high investment and deep involvement in the day-to-day routines of children's lives.[22] Sociologist Annette Lareau's comparative research on parental involvement found that while working-class parents were more likely to defer to the judgments about their child made by school officials such as teachers and guidance counselors, seeing them as having a distinct professional expertise, upper-middle-class professional parents rarely did. Instead, they were highly interventionist, which many sociologists attribute to rising anxiety about the reproduction of social class advantage and fear about their children's possible downward mobility.[23] As Lareau notes, the consequence is that children of professional, middle-class parents, as they watch by example, learn to advocate for themselves in institutional settings and develop an emerging sense of entitlement to services and opportunities within school and beyond.

The Rise of Organic Snacking

With some exceptions, Washington parents hail from a new class of worker, highly educated, intellectual laborers, social and cultural specialists for whom food, just like academics, carries tremendous cultural importance and is the subject of significant consideration. Sociologist Michele Lamont argues that for this segment of the upper-middle class, "[B]ecause their professional energies . . . are oriented toward attaining cultural, spiritual, humanitarian goals, and because their professional achievement cannot be measured primarily in economic terms, one can expect these people to put more emphasis on cultural and moral standards of evaluation."[24] Here again we see how food carries considerable symbolic importance. "Food cultures" and food itself have long been recognized as tied to both class habitus, the distinct set of embodied dispositions that pattern our tastes and preferences, and cultural capital, that is, the cultural knowledge that shapes the way we render judgments about cultural goods. Habitus and cultural capital, taken together, materialize into specific cultural practices and aesthetic dispositions that over time become expressive resources through which to project cultural and class identity, but in a way that is so routine, it is all but taken for granted.[25] Internalized and embodied, these class sensibilities, or class logics, help to explain why we feel repelled by some food choices and not others—favoring Chipotle but not McDonald's, sushi but not fish sticks. In this distinct way, food is a meaningful cultural resource that at once expresses a distinct set of class dispositions but also serves to embed them into school life. Food, even the much-maligned school food, is taken up as a basis to signal class distinction, a means by which the school was able to project a distinct identity as a public school serving a select segment of the general population—in other words, not your average public school.

In the late French sociologist Pierre Bourdieu's formulation of the cultural dimensions of class, aesthetics, restraint, and form were pivotal categories around which class disposition structured the field of food consumption. Eating constitutes a cultural repertoire that involves "high status signals" in which "ordinary choices of everyday existence revealing deep rooted, long standing dispositions" are expressed.[26] For Bourdieu, the whole constellation of activity that is involved in eating (manners, food selection, portion size, appreciation of and judgment about food) expresses our cultural capital, our social position, and our class habitus. This, I submit, had profound impact on the school cafeteria and the food it served at Washington.

This was expressed in the parental involvement that led to the school district deciding to hire a new food director who could better align school food with professional, middle-class health concerns in the first place. The two vending machines in the cafeteria provide a particularly rich example. They were regularly stocked with a bevy of processed food and drink items that belong to an upscale market used to signal social distinction. They are foods we might find at Whole Foods or Trader Joe's, but not likely at Wal-Mart.[27] Drinks included San Pellegrino sparkling juice, Horizon organic chocolate milk, and Honest Kids. Snacks included Clif Bars, Smartfood popcorn, Hippie chips (baked chips), Stacy's pita chips, and Kashi fruit bars.[28] These food items belong to a category of consumption we often associate with "healthy" eating, thought to be good for the body and long-term health, and express the array of morally acceptable snacks for what sociologists recognize as the newly emerged idealized child figure, "the organic child," whose food choices, often made for them, protect against environmental and health risks associated with an industrial food system.[29] The remarks of Lia, Karen, and Chelsea, a group of friends from Washington, are revealing:

> LIA: They took out all of the candy machines, all of the soda machines
> KAREN: And replaced it with healthy stuff.
> LIA: Soy wafers, oh my god!
> KAREN: Water.
> CHANTAL: Organic graham crackers.
> KAREN: Pita chips.
> CHELSEA: Healthy stuff, they really cracked down on it.
> LIA: They turned into Trader Joe's . . .

These are snack foods that are likely to be found in the kitchen cupboards of many of these students, and in this sense, the vending machine reflects a particular set of consumer sensibilities held by parents, which also helps to explain why the vending machines stirred such significant comment from both students and parents, as Dan had earlier remarked. Thus, lunchroom food at Washington reflected efforts to approximate foods found at home, and in the process contributed to the sedimentation of a moral order whereby the private is cast as superior to the public. This contrasts to Thurgood, where the food served was often seen as a corrective to home-based foods.[30] This, I suggest, represents a broader orientation to school as a public institution, whereby the morally privileged sites of social life reside not within our public institutions but outside them, often making our collective and individual investments in them difficult to sustain over time (and as we will see, resulting in disengagement by those with the resources to opt out altogether).

These are snack foods often associated with what sociologists have identified as moral or ethical consumption, signaling an *aesthetic orientation to health*, or *food philosophy*, a point of contention for Brenda, Thurgood's food director, as readers may recall. These snack foods carry distinctive signs about the bearer—often superficially communicating upper-middle-class parenting styles of care, something Doritos and Cheetos fail to communicate. Lia's comment about Trader Joe's is especially poignant since Trader Joe's, like Whole Foods (sometimes called "Whole Paycheck"), is often associated with gentrification in neighborhoods and the displacement of lower-income residents, which also raises questions about moral and ethical consumption.

These snack foods belong to what market insiders call "snacking and impulse food markets," "where quality seeking" ranks highest among the consumer. For this set of consumers, marketers realized, "Snacking products based around quality ingredients, hand craftsmanship, and authenticity will be well placed," according to a recent food marketing research report.[31] Sociologists Johnston and Baumann have identified simplicity and authenticity as core culinary virtues defining the contemporary gourmet foodscape. Undeniably, school food exists well outside the gourmet food landscape, yet the call for food change by parents in the Washington school community expresses some of the same culinary virtues, epitomized by the names of commercial snack brands such as "Honest Kids" and "Smartfood."

Here we can also identify a distinctly class-based orientation to health, what Bourdieu once called "the cult of health," where aesthetic concerns, that is, lifestyle and tastes, are difficult to disentangle from actual nutritional health and out of which a "moralized class hierarchy" is produced and reproduced.[32] As Bourdieu argues in his seminal *Distinction*, "The body is the most indisputable materialization of class taste." Here he is speaking to how class patterns the way of managing the body, "a way of treating it, caring for it, feeding it and maintaining it."[33] Of course, the idea of "healthy" processed food seems an oxymoron. Perhaps they are better than other snack foods made with high fructose corn syrup or trans fats, but they still are processed foods, high in sodium and fillers with little nutritional value. Yet, they tend to be treated as morally superior, cast against less pure junk foods like Doritos and Oreos. Upper-middle-class parents have the resources to buy these foods and the power to compel schools to offer them. For Dan, his work was fundamentally about negotiating these parental demands, thereby making the food choices appealing to parents.

"It's Not High-Quality Ice Cream, but It's Okay"

Ultimately, Dan had to satisfy the students who consumed these foods, a group who shared the same class sensibilities held by their parents but who also often rejected parental food choices and embraced youth food sensibilities that circulate in a broader discursive context that defines adolescent food choices as being fundamentally at odds with health-oriented adult food choices. Some prided themselves on food choices that cut against the grain; others' choices were squarely within the familiar round of adolescent food preferences. Complaints about school food, though not frequent, served as one such manifestation of the tussle between adolescents and adults.[34] Some complaints seemed a genuine and spontaneous response to the lunch offered, as in the case of one boy who was standing in the lunch line at Washington and after reviewing the lunch offerings announced, though to no one in particular, "I'm not getting anything." Other complaints seemed more purposeful—used instead toward social ends as a means to express discontent with something more substantial at school. When uttered publicly, food complaints signified more than just dissatisfaction with food but occupied part of a continuum of food talk that helped to constitute the distinct social fabric of the space and the youth within it. There is a performative dimension to food complaints and food refusals enacted by youth that expresses both young people's negotiation within school and peer groups and their alignment with youth cultural groups. A publicly declared lament operates as a means to position oneself before a crowd. I can recall on one occasion watching as a girl declared loudly and with much bravado, "It's disgusting!" as she pushed her tray to the center of the table with a look of deep disdain as other kids at the table leaned in and tried what she had rejected (a pulled-pork sandwich). Food complaints are similar then to what anthropologist Mimi Nichter has called "fat talk," in that they too have a rapport-building function. Collective complaints can serve as a means to express group membership—consider the comment made by one student: "What kind of malarkey are *they* serving *us* today?" This is perhaps especially meaningful from a developmental standpoint since early high school is a key period in the formation of social identity and sense of group position. When I began this research, I expected kids' complaints to be tied to dignity and self-worth, and thus hypothesized that food complaints would be much more numerous at Thurgood, a school with a larger percentage of lower-income students often denied dignity of self in school. Instead I found the opposite to be true. Food complaints were more common at Washington and almost nonexistent at Thurgood. This, I suggest, can be explained in part by the complex relationship upper-income kids form to school as a public institution and arises from the tension between democratic ideology and status distinction that public schools in upper-income communities come to represent as simultaneously exclusive and open and meritocratic.[35] The tension between these two opposing frames gives way to a posture of ambivalence by upper-income youth, shaping the way they relate to school food and a public food provisioning system, and also places enormous pressure on administrators in these schools to continually distance themselves from other public schools, while also fulfilling the democratic mandate of broad access that is the fundamental mission of public schools.

While I observed public repudiations of school food, even more common were food evaluations, willingly and regularly offered by youth at Washington, again almost entirely absent in Thurgood. Like food complaints, food evaluations express dispositions and expectations toward food and enable the display of cultural and moral judgments, which is generally recognized among sociologists as central to the work of class distinction and thus part of the identity work and the performance of self. On one occasion, two Washington boys came in, assessing the scene and selection. One paused for a moment before saying, "I think that's the safest bet" as he pointed to the steak sandwich. On another occasion a young woman who had been eating her lunch alone approached me as she prepared to exit the lunchroom. "Can I ask what you are doing?" I told her I was studying the cafeteria and she replied, "Well, if you're going to eat the food, may I suggest you go for the potato. You will be much better off."[36]

An emergent food consciousness was easy to identify among students at Washington, and in this sense, the cafeteria reflected a distinct, class-based aesthetic and style of cultural consumption that was given expression in the way the larger population of students related to school food. From my first visits, signs of professional, middle-class life were numerous, embedded in objects—what Bourdieu called "external signs"[37]—

that were easily recognizable as part of the adolescent cultural life of the professional middle class. I saw more than a smattering of Vera Bradley bags, Tom's shoes, and Whole Foods brown paper bags, metal bottles for water, and college t-shirts with logos from elite universities—Princeton, Northwestern, Stanford, and Yale—worn by many kids.[38] Students' evaluation of the food served often assumed a distinct class tone, reflective of their expectations about food quality and form, and the sense of entitlement to good food they held was homologous to their class position. I can recall standing in line, watching as kids moved through the lunch, when a girl turned to her friend as she picked up a small container of ice cream from the freezer and remarked in a tone of utter seriousness, "It's not high-quality ice cream, but it's okay." Thus, just as parents' evaluations were influential in the way Dan addressed matters of health and diet and food's appeal, as discussed earlier, so too were students'.

The emerging sense of entitlement sociologist Annette Lareau identifies with the professional middle class was expressed in the types of requests students made and also shaped the scope of food offerings. While they were virtually absent at Thurgood, at Washington I witnessed regular requests by students for modification and personalized accommodations as I stood in line beside them. Students moved through the lunch lines, making various requests: "two egg rolls" instead of the standard one; "only one biscuit, no chicken"; "a biscuit, but no rice"; "just chicken." I witnessed requests for food that wasn't even on the food line. In one instance, a boy who spotted pizza on a rack several feet behind the food service workers asked, "Can I have that back there?" In another, I overheard a girl say to a friend, "I'm going to see if they have the wrap." And in another, I watched as two girls moved into line and one of the girls asked if they had any more ham sandwiches. In a last case, another boy came in, asked for nuggets, and was told "no more" by one of the food service workers. "Don't you have some in the back?" he asked, but was again told no by the same worker. He persisted, "Can I have some of that pizza, then?"—although the pizza was also not on the food line but on a tray behind the food worker. These requests certainly kept the food service workers on their toes and the pace of their work continuous, allowing little break in the line. Honoring these individual requests for modification produced greater demand and burden for the food service workers, while also reproducing a sense of entitlement as students came to expect personal accommodations in institutional settings. This entitlement is recognized as central to the reproduction of class privilege and a defining aspect of the way upper-income groups make use of public institutions more generally, bending them to their will rather than the other way around.[39]

Passing the Time, Food Play, and Food Antics

School food holds little if any sacred value—certainly not in the way home-made food eaten with family does. It is institutional, mass produced for public consumption, and stripped of its emotional value for the students who consume it. Little care is afforded to school food. It is tossed around, thrown in the trash, eaten without comment—which helps to explain why school food can become an object of play. The folklorist Anna Berensin advances the notion of play as expressive culture, arguing that play is a site where a broad range of cultural narratives are worked through. So what does play in this context express? I suggest that food play is part of youth's public culture and expresses young people's indifference to school food as a public good, and that class is a central mediator of this indifference. At Washington, food play was a means to pass the time, to constitute the boundaries of groups, and to confirm friendships, on the one hand, but also a means to express ambivalence toward *public* school. Arguably, this was helped along by the fact that few kids appeared to need a full thirty minutes to eat lunch; the last ten minutes were largely social, with kids playing cards or fiddling with their iPods and phones. I watched as boys stacked empty milk containers and attempted to build models from contorted plastic forks. At one lunch I watched two boys at a table of about ten boys play what looked like a game of hot potato with a sandwich bag that held what was now a very flat sandwich. One boy tossed it to the other and it fell to the ground with a splat. The boy eventually leaned down to pick it up and tossed it to the other boy, who pretended to toss it into the garbage but in the end kept it in his hand and exited the room. I watched kids mix foods together, pretzels and apple sauce, for instance. "I dare you to eat this," one girl challenged those at her table, but there were no takers. Kids playfully pretended to shove food into each other's mouths and pretended to throw small milk cartons, apples, and other food items at each other. In a few instances, food was tossed though not actually thrown, and all was relatively calm. The antics were minor affairs, small pranks. A single bottle of chocolate milk sat upside down, balancing without a cap, for example. "We have a prank here," announced the principal, calling it for what it was. He turned and advised the lunch lady to be careful when she cleaned it up, and in one quick swoop she picked up the bottle and covered the top with her hand. A small amount of milk spilled out. She smiled, as did I, since she prevented what could have been a bigger mess, but the event ended before it even started, and another lunch began.

This type of food play is a limited liability action for these youth. They can express indifference to school lunch without running the risk of any real trouble that might undermine their future mobility, and at the same time render visible the boredom that characterizes much of school.[40] On the surface of things (at least at school), Washington students' behavior largely aligned with the expectations held by the middle-class professional adults who governed them. I remember on my first visit to the school, meeting one of the teachers in the cafeteria. At both Thurgood and Washington, since I was an unknown adult, teachers I had not met passing through the cafeteria always approached me to confirm my purpose in being there. On this day, I was approached by a teacher; I told him about the project, my interest in what kids eat and do during school lunch, and he immediately replied, "These are good kids," adding, "No problems." "These are good kids" is a statement I came to hear from virtually every single adult I encountered at Washington: the principal, the security staff, teachers, the food director. During my first week at Washington, Joe remarked, "It's different here. You'll see. Even the so-called bad kids aren't that bad." "Harmless," he added. "Maybe 5 percent bad apples, ten kids who are trouble." The "good kids" mantra, as I came to think of it, hinted that the standard default kid is not good, that their school is the exception. This mindset was so pervasive, it was impossible to think of it as anything other than a broader institutional orientation. But youth scholars have complicated this picture, showing how "good kids" are kids who on the surface of things hover below the radar of trouble. They appear clean-cut, future oriented, and academically focused, even while pursuing youth cultural ends outside the purview of adults. These are the kids whose outward appearance and demeanor suggest acceptance of the definition of school articulated by the administration and teachers, what Penelope Eckert identified as kids whose behaviors are well aligned with the corporate logic of school. For these kids, their demeanor reflects professional, middle-class, adolescent scripts of public behavior that the kids at Thurgood, with the exception of the AP kids, were less likely to follow, as readers may recall. The consequence is two different trajectories through school, two different encounters with this public institution, including its lunchroom.

Commercial Food and the Gift Economy of Youth

Unlike school food, which is a symbol of the banal culture of public institutions, commercial food represents a break with boredom. That is its very promise and why it is so coveted in school. Thus, understanding kids' relationships to food in school means understanding their relationship to school. I remember, about a month into my observations at Washington, arriving to a lunch scene with two long lunch lines with kids excitedly chatting. What was the source of their excitement? Domino's pizza for lunch, left over from the annual schoolwide picnic in honor of retiring staff and teachers held the day before. I watched as kids began to trickle in as the lunch ladies were furiously trying to plate the pizza for kids to take. "Oh my god!" a brown-haired boy in shorts and a Princeton t-shirt loudly screeched, "Is that pizza?" as he looked around at the other kids in line and then back at the pizza. He held in his hand a crumpled-up brown bag, presumably his lunch brought from home. He was exuberant. "Domino's! It's Domino's! . . . It's been like two months." He looked at his lunch bag again and turned quickly on his heels toward a table as he tried to unload it. He found no takers. Kids came in and in rapid succession grabbed tray after tray of pizza. It was a controlled chaos. There were no takers for the pork barbeque or lasagna, also on the menu. I overheard, "Peeeezzzza." I walked around the lunch room and noted that every student in the room who had purchased lunch had pizza, except one. Pizza, a once-weekly staple food item prior to Dan's arrival, was now offered every few weeks. This pizza was doubly special because it was Domino's, a commercial pizza and not your run-of-the-mill school pizza that high schoolers from various schools tell me usually requires a paper napkin to absorb the excess grease.

More common were commercial foods that were brought by students themselves, with the purpose of being shared with friends as a means to construct a collective encounter. Many students, because of family resources, moved easily within consumer markets, using their disposable income to introduce high-demand, high-status foods into school and thus gain recognition among peers through food in a way that was not in evidence at Thurgood because of a lack of disposable income to do so. During one Washington lunch, as the kids filtered in and out of line, I caught a girl with large, round, dark-rimmed glasses and a short pixie haircut, who hopped out of the line with a tin of Pepperidge Farm cookies visibly displayed in her arm. In the course of lunch, I watched as she shared her cookies with those around her, gaining recognition and acknowledgment from others. At another lunch, I watched a boy whip out a bag of Keebler chocolate chip cookies. With a smile registered on his face, he displayed the bag for his friends to see, signaling the promise of sharing later.

Outside food draws public attention and the inevitable request, "Can I have one?" and in this sense, commercial food serves as a visible prop facilitating particular types of exchanges. Whether commercial foods, from Keebler chocolate chip cookies to sushi, were willingly offered as a gift, begrudgingly shared, or withheld signaled a public acknowledgment of friendship, on the one hand, and the enactment of status rituals, on the other. Commercial foods, in this sense, are central to the gift economy of youth, in a way school food will never be.[41] Commercial market foods in school, then, serve social ends above anything else. I can recall during one lunch a boy handed a girl a can of Coke. She looked at it with eyebrows raised and a coy tilt of her head and asked, "For me?" and then matter-of-factly told the boy she didn't really want it. Another girl came in and he extended the Coke to her. Her eyes lit up. "Really?" she asked, and then accepted the offering with an open display of appreciation for the unexpected gift, perhaps made all the more meaningful because it was food gifted by a boy to a girl. I witnessed very few instances of food gifting from a boy to a girl at either school or fast-food places, especially when compared to the number of times I observed girls gift food to boys. Recall the requests by boys to girls to gift their free or reduced lunch noted in the last chapter. I also observed instances when girls' requests to boys for the gift of food were rejected outright, which suggests that status rituals around food gifting are tied to gender in adolescent worlds.

Commercial food is prized and usually seized as an object for sharing and gifting. But commercial foods were not gifted to just anyone. In many cases, I watched others lobby the student in possession of the outside food until the student grudgingly caved, submitting to the litany of requests.[42] Foods were shared with close friends and usually status equals. As I already mentioned, girls were usually the ones to offer the gift of food. I watched girls bring cupcakes, bags of candy, popcorn, and chips, all brought with the intent to be shared. On one occasion, I watched as a girl proudly held in her hand a large AriZona iced tea and a bag of Doritos and the girls at the table cheered. At another lunch, I observed a table of girls host a mini–birthday party, replete with a giant Mrs. Fields chocolate chip cookie trimmed with red icing.[43] In many ways, this is not surprising. Plenty of research has demonstrated how deeply invested girls are in relationships and the sense of self they derive from the bonds of friendships formed through the sharing of food, clothes, and make-up.[44]

Kids rarely, if ever, shared lunch bought from school.[45] Since school lunch is available to all, it provides little opportunity to forge or signal what Erving Goffman called "tie signs," public displays that "contain evidence" about the intensity and intimacy of particular social relationships.[46] Some foods lend themselves to easy sharing. A smoothie, for example, requires a more intimate form of sharing than does a bag of popcorn. Body contact is implied since lips are likely to grace the same straw, and thus such foods communicate what Goffman called the "I'm with" affiliation. In these forms of sharing, ideas about contamination of the body hover just above the surface of the interaction.[47] Anthropologist Mary Douglas, well known for her examination of the symbolic boundaries that separate objects as either sacred or polluted, would probably regard these exchanges as negotiations around status.[48] Certain bodies threaten to pollute others and thus distance and avoidance are important, especially since food is such a significant tie sign, bound to status displays.[49]

The expectation of sharing can also serve as a source of conflict, however. On one occasion I watched a group squabble over a small bag of fruity snacks that had been purchased from the vending machine. "I gave you some last time," I heard one boy protest, to which the boy sitting next to him retorted, "You are all taking like handfuls!" At this, a third boy got up, walked over to the machine, and purchased his own fruity snacks. In this instance, the matter is not about a shortage of money to replenish the supply of fruity snacks, but a tussle over friendship norms about entitlements and obligations.[50] During another lunch I overheard a boy declare, "I have no money," as he turned and threw himself at a table, landing in a chair. He was performing a type of desperate hunger with his body as it convulsed in the chair, his hand gripping his stomach. His friends looked at him, unpersuaded, as they continued to eat their lunch. One of them shook his head, as if in an emphatic, "No way." I heard the hungry boy say to one of the other guys at the table, "I have no money," and the boy responded, "Dude, I don't have any money either," as he took a sip from his soda bottle, eating his small bag of chips. Another guy next to him offered an unsympathetic, "No way." Finally, one of the boys took a small handful of potato chips and placed them on the table next to his tray for the boy to eat, separating the gift of food from his own supply, presumably to prevent the boy from eating freely off his own tray. I left with the sense that this may have been a familiar scene for these friends, and in this instance, the sanction served to clarify friendship norms around sharing.

Conclusion

Unlike family food, school food holds little if any sacred value; nor does it contain the allure of commercial foods. Commercial foods represent the world beyond the confines of school. This was most apparent at Washington since only a small portion of students qualify for free or reduced lunch, and thus the types of food are more varied. What is clear is that for some kids, school lunch will continue to be regarded with indifference (and in some cases open contempt). That is the case because the food is school food. In principle, kids find the relationship to public school objectionable, not the food itself (even though some school food really does warrant genuine complaint). Boredom with food is also about boredom with school. Lunch is a break from academic routines, whereas market foods signify a break in the day and serve as a reminder of a commercial life cast as infinitely more interesting than school.[51]

Unlike in the commercial realm where options (Panera, Chipotle, Taco Bell, Baja Fresh) appear limitless, with food choice depending entirely on what someone is in the mood for, in school, by comparison, even at a place like Thurgood, which can boast twenty meal offerings daily, the range of options narrows significantly. The issue of boredom with food is difficult to get around in institutional settings of a large scale where budget constraints are felt daily, where boredom itself often knocks at the proverbial door. Yet at the same time, much of this is bundled up with the way we think about public institutions and the goods and services that are offered within them, including the food.

Class plays an important role in the social organization of school lunch and its food.[52] As a public good, school food is an object of indifference for kids in upper-income communities, many of whom can easily opt out of school lunch or transform it into an object of limited liability play. Class dispositions were also reflected in the way students at Washington evaluated school foods while also giving rise to parental pressure to transform what was on the menu. For Dan, managing parents was a fundamental part of his work, consuming his time and energy as he sought to make changes that would satisfy parents and kids alike. As Dan noted, many of the kids were slow to change, openly lamenting the loss of daily french fries, ice cream, and pizza on Fridays, high-demand items in youth worlds, while parents called for rapid change. Parental and student expectations of particular types of food directed many of the choices Dan made, and managing parental complaints and doing preemptive PR work represented a core dimension of his job.

Meaningfully, these class dynamics set in motion Dan's decision in 2013 to no longer participate in the National School Lunch Program. Parents and students together played a significant role in the decision to leave the NSLP. Without a high percentage of kids on free and reduced lunch, combined with the large number of kids who could easily opt out of lunch, students' participation in the NSLP was low. For Dan, leaving NSLP enabled him to better satisfy student demand, adjust portion size, reduce food waste, do more on-site cooking, and introduce more healthy food items better aligned with parental demand. While the cost of lunch for students increased by almost a dollar, student participation increased dramatically. Longer lunch lines, because of greater student participation, became the cause of student complaint. But during the period of time I observed in 2010, before Dan left the NSLP, food was used for symbolic ends: a means of play, to pass the time, and in some cases to comment on school.

The decision to leave the NSLP means that this school has left behind a broad-based public food provisioning system serving schools in poor, middle-income, and upper-income communities. The defection of those with substantial resources from public institutions in the end weakens those institutions, while their sustained investment in them creates the conditions to improve them. The cases of Washington High School and Thurgood High School illustrate the promise of a public food provisioning system to promote dietary health for all, but also its limits, capturing the dilemmas and struggle of public institutions in a context of deepening inequalities between and within communities across the United States.

5

I'm Lovin' It

Fast Food and After-School Hot Spots

I need a double cheeseburger and hold the lettuce
Don't be frontin son, no seeds on a bun
We be up in this
Drive thru
Order for two
I gots a craving for a number 9 like my
Shoe
We need some chicken up in here
In this dizzle,
For rizzle, my nizzle
Extra salt on the frizzle
Dr. Pepper my brother
Another for your mother
Double, double, super size
And don't forget the FRIES
—Big Mac rap

We be up in Wendy's doing
what taste right
I'll be lookin at the menu, I'll be here all night.
So I'll start off with one of em
Kid's meal, but with no pickles on the burger baby, let's keep it real
I've got more rhymes than Wendy's got orders and you
Be hearing this right now, wishing you had a recorder
to complete my order. What you got for side dishes?
Mmm, girl, second thought
hook me up with fried fishes
Mmm a garden salad we'll go,
need that for show
You aint' gotta ask it ain't for
Here, it's to go.
—Wendy's rap

These are drive-through raps, and they are wildly popular. Set to the syncopation of a human beat-box and performed by young men as they move through the drive-through, this sort of rhyming and free-styling is video recorded, usually by a friend also in the car, and then later uploaded to YouTube, where it is archived alongside innumerable other raps that are available for public viewing. Part adolescent prank, part creative youth digital expression, these fast-food raps for Burger King, Taco Bell, Arby's, and, of course, the ubiquitous McDonald's enable youth to stake a claim in public life and to gain visibility in a world where the boundaries between the virtual and real, as well as the public and private, realms of social existence lack clear demarcation.

In 2013, several years after the first fast-food rap was uploaded to the internet, the funk rapper Mr B., a white college kid, rapped his order, set to music, into the intercom at a Wendy's as he sat behind the wheel while a friend recorded his performance. The employee on the other end of the intercom got the order exactly as requested, which included four small Sprites and a ten-piece order of chicken tenders, and then "comped" the order. Whether this was a planned, scripted, or spontaneous action, within days, the video had gone viral.

Even the decidedly suburban Starbucks has inspired drive-through raps. In one YouTube video, a white teenage girl identified as "Vanilla Latte" and her sidekick, "the Tall Frothy one," rapped about scones, chai tea, Frappaccino, and Caramel Macchiato. The rap was taken as an expression of good-natured fun by the Starbucks worker on the other end of the intercom, as the girl who performed the rap explained that they wrote their rap in "calculus class." In another rap uploaded to YouTube, the food service worker on the other end of the intercom actually raps back the order—and again the meal is offered at no expense.

These raps are in principle about play. The rhyming is silly and intended for a laugh, and there is the expectation of a favorable response of some kind from the person on the other end of the intercom, although exceptions do occur. In 2009, four Utah teenagers met a much less desirable fate and were arrested for rapping their order at a McDonald's drive-through and then cited for disorderly conduct, even though they promptly left the McDonald's when asked to do so by the worker. The reception of "drive-through raps" has been uneven, interpreted in this case as a prank gone too far, and in this sense, these raps also capture the precarious place of youth in public space. Yet, at the same time, commercial markets, motivated by the promise of increased profit margins and greater market share among youth, often co-opt these creative expressions arising from the everyday worlds of youth. That Taco Bell capitalized on this youth-based, home-grown creative production and produced its own "drive-through rap" commercial to promote its eighty-nine-cent chicken burrito provides one example of the all-too-common commercial appropriation of youth culture for market ends.

The global currency of hip-hop in the broader mainstream youth culture helps to explain the draw of the beat-box and free-styling over country twang or some other musical form.[1] There is also something significant about the fact that the fast-food drive-through, rather than some other cultural space, is seized as the object of play, the location for what cultural studies scholar Paul Willis has termed youth's "symbolic work."[2] The folklorist Anna Beresin observes, "[S]ymbolic work and creativity place identities in larger wholes. . . . [S]ymbolic work and creativity develop and affirm our active sense of our own vital capacities, the power of the self and how they might be applied to the cultural world."[3]

That fast food would be absorbed into youth cultural production is much less curious when one considers the amount of time kids spend in commercial fast-food settings after school and on weekends with family and friends and the sheer ubiquity of fast food even in noncommercial spaces. Commercial food markets have long played an important role in mediating the meaning of youth food consumption, shaping the types of food youth are likely to consume and the meanings they assign to that food.[4] Paul, a first-year student at a local community college, declared, "I love Burger King! I kind of grew up on fast food. I love fast food. I probably, before I came to college, I probably went and got fast food two to three times a week." Another college student echoed this same sentiment: "I'm all about Taco Bell." The convenience of fast food carried significant appeal for both the high school– and the college-aged youth I interviewed across class groups. "It's really fast, you walk in, you walk out. It's a good price." For higher-income kids, Panera, Cheesecake Factory, Chipotle, and Elevation Burger usually made their short list, replacing McDonald's and Taco Bell but not fast food itself. The symbolic worlds of youth are hard to disentangle from commodity culture. In this sense, drive-through raps can be understood as symptomatic of the commercial market's hold over youth *and* youth's creative engagement and influence over those very markets. And thus, drive-through raps both capture and reflect the contradictory relationship youth form to commercial markets today.

Meaning and Markets: The After-School Rush

What is the draw of fast food for young people? Sure, the appeal of fast food can certainly be explained by the fact that it's rich in salt and fat; those french fries from McDonald's really do taste good.[5] Such an explanation, as valid as it is, in the end fails to help us better understand the complicated and contradictory connections between markets and meaning and their relationship to other spheres of social existence. Meaning matters. When McDonald's opened its first store over two decades ago in France, French officials expected it to fail, seeing it largely as the "menace of Americanization," standardization, and "cheap commercialism." But it was a hit, at least among French teens. The freedom from adult supervision, self-service, and its aesthetic made it a successful alternative to "stuffy" French restaurants.[6] In Beijing, McDonald's is only affordable for the upwardly mobile, urban middle class, yet for its youth, McDonald's represents "the modern."[7] Of course, fast food doesn't appeal exclusively to young people. Adults are daily consumers of fast food.[8] The difference, however, lies in the extent to which fast food is adopted for youth cultural ends, which is the subject of this chapter.

In the United States, consumption of fast food is a main avenue through which American youth gain access to public life and the commercial world, since food as a commodity is relatively inexpensive. Their money buys them access, allowing them to linger if they choose. And thus, fast food signifies membership and participation in community life. This has long been the case. Recall the nostalgic Rockwellian images of white, middle-class, suburban kids clustered around the soda counters during the postwar period, a period marked by the expansion of a middle class, rapid suburbanization, and the migration of leisure activities into a quasi-public commercial realm that was enabled by the rise of discretionary income by mostly white, middle-class parents and their children. The experience of teens of color requires a different historical accounting, since segregation in commercial spaces was still enabled by law; work and leisure patterns for communities of color were less likely to unfold in commercial realms; discretionary income was lower because wages remained much lower; and entry to the suburbs remained blocked.[9]

But before going further with this line of reasoning, it is useful to distinguish among fast foods (not all are created equally, after all) and the places where we eat. In other words, we should separate the cultural object from the cultural scene. In my time observing at fast-food outlets over the last several years, I observed many young people order their food and take it "to go," suggesting the obvious—little importance is attached to the fast-food setting itself. However, I saw many more stay, lingering in booths and tables, seizing the area as a space of sociability. As Karla explains, referring to Taco Bell, "It's like the place where everyone comes to meet. Like, if you go there, there's going to be someone that you know there, all the time." For youth, these settings are the "Great Good Places" sociologist Ray Oldenburg identifies as being fundamental to informal public life.[10]

Oldenburg's "Great Good Places" has relevance for understanding the period directly following the end of the school day, what I've been calling the "postschool rush."[11] This is the period of time when young people are most likely to linger in fast-food outlets in groups, thereby transforming commercial settings into something else—*youth cultural scenes.* But why do some public food places emerge as vibrant youth enclaves, what Oldenburg calls "third places" beyond school and home, and others do not? This chapter examines youth's public food consumption in commercial fast-food settings in answer to that question. It focuses on the emotional charge of what the sociologist Erving Goffman famously characterized as "the situation" to understand the pull of fast-food settings for youth, over and above the food itself.[12]

As with the previous chapters, this chapter highlights the symbolic realm through which meaning is created in an effort to understand what inspires action. Focusing on food consumption as it comes into being through collective activities, the broader aim of this chapter is to illuminate the cultural and situational dimensions of youth commercial food consumption to decenter the individual food consumer, too often taken as the starting point in health policies promoting behavioral change.[13] In focusing on the situational and the collective, I also avoid treating action and meaning as expressions of the macro-structure of consumer food markets that is too often assumed in discussions of youth and food markets, which is especially apparent in discussions of deceptive advertising. Social science research has demonstrated growing youth cynicism toward marketing, which speaks to the complicated relationship youth forge to consumer markets.[14] I examine instead the process and micro-structure of the situation itself as guide for action.[15] As Goffman argued long ago, "situations" are rarely recognized for their structuring influence in their own right; as a result, the structure of social encounters is rarely given its full due.[16] Yet attention to these situational dimensions of fast-food scenes helps us to understand why teens return to fast-food settings day after day. These cultural scenes, generated through performance and play, are where kids access a public youth community and participate in symbolic exchanges, in the form of gift giving of food, that solidify group boundaries and membership. In the process, their actions serve to project a collectively anchored youth identity, set against identities belonging to adult worlds.

Whether a fast-food restaurant is transformed into a youth cultural scene depends on a number of variables. Not all McDonald's restaurants emerge or endure as youth cultural scenes, for example. In the four McDonald's restaurants where I observed after school, youth participation was uneven. At the McDonald's across the street from Washington High, a community where the median home price is $630,000, the base of customers was largely elderly Asian and South American immigrants, not kids.[17] While few kids were found at this McDonald's, they could be found scattered at Starbucks, Elevation Burger, Robeks, and Chipotle, all considerably more upscale fast-food establishments, and all also within a close walk of school. Importantly, all are better aligned with meanings about health and food quality that have become an important expression of upper-middle-class identity. At the McDonald's across the street from Edwards High School, the place was usually packed with kids. Importantly, McDonald's was the *only* commercial food outlet that could be accessed easily on foot by these students after school. The McDonald's restaurants down the street from Thurgood and Hampton high schools were also often packed with kids.

Just around the Corner

I often joke that if you want to find a McDonald's, all you have to do is find a high school. In cities and suburbs across the United States, McDonald's stores are often a short walk from nearby high schools. Apparently this can't be chalked up entirely to coincidence, but instead reflects efforts to increase youth's market participation by shaping the food environment near schools.[18] Thus, high schools, by default, serve as feeders to commercial food hot spots. This was the case for the McDonald's restaurants I observed. All were within a block of school and all—with the exception of one McDonald's where the base of customers was largely elderly Asian and South American immigrants, as I already mentioned—were popular after-school destinations for high school students not yet eligible to drive. Most of the young people I talked to preferred the taste of Chipotle, for example, to McDonald's, yet McDonald's was far and away the more popular postschool destination. Students return to McDonald's daily. Kids go to McDonald's because it is cheap and close to school. Access is given freely with minimum purchase, and in some instances none at all. Subway, for example, which is a few stores up in the same strip mall across the street from Hampton High, is double in price for the same amount of food. "Too expensive!" a group of boys explained to me one afternoon as we sat eating french fries at McDonald's. Chipotle, while uniformly characterized as delicious, was also thought to be "a rip" as one girl remarked to me, "I'll go there when I want to spend eight dollars on a burrito!" In this specific way, money and mobility help to determine the mix of participants at these settings, as does a meaning system that sorts fast food on a value scale. "When I go out, I don't want to go to McDonald's, I want something good," Ashley, an upper-income high schooler explained. "Some of the guys in our group go to Burger King, but I don't care for it," echoed Chelsea, Ashley's best friend. "It's kind of dirty." To the increasingly health-conscious youth residing in upper-income areas in the United States, McDonald's represents a stigmatized and debased consumption, that is, poor food for poor folks. It was eaten only as a last resort. As one girl from Washington High School told me, "I mean we have like McDonald's and Burger King but we never go there." "I'm used to eating like healthier things I guess," offered another girl, also from Washington

High School. "I mean McDonald's and Wendy's? I can't imagine the last time I've eaten anything from there. Sushi or a Panera salad will sound more appealing."[19] Enduring links between gender and food filter these class meanings such that boys across class groups could justify their fast-food choice on the simple grounds "Gotta eat," where for upper-income girls the forces of class and gender conspire to constrain choice.[20]

In contrast, for kids living in high-poverty urban communities where access to healthy foods is severely constrained, McDonald's was seen as a better alternative to the run-down corner stores where candy, soda, and chips were usually bought in large quantities before and after school. At one urban school I visited, many kids would have welcomed a McDonald's across the street from their school, rather than the abandoned lot littered with empty beer cans, Dorito bags, and cigarette butts. There were no fast-food places where you could sit for any period of time, consigning youth to the streets, but there was plenty of take-out, and a long line of kids extended out the door of the corner convenience store across from school each morning before school and each afternoon. In this way, community-based inequalities remain meaningful to young people's consumer experiences, even if not in the guise of deliberate exclusion.[21]

The four McDonald's restaurants I observed are all located in ethnically and class-diverse, resource-rich counties, not poor ones, and are part of a major metropolitan area. At Hampton High, across the street from the McDonald's I visited the most, the base of students is ethnically mixed and tends toward the middle class, with a large number of military families and midlevel professionals.[22] Yet, while the school is ethnically mixed, McDonald's is not. It is largely a space dominated by black and brown JV and third-string footballers and basketballers and the cheer squad; most are freshmen and sophomores, mouths brimming with braces, and none have cars; boys outnumber girls.[23] (Sports participation, which is patterned by race, largely predicts who frequents this McDonald's.) Edwards and Thurgood are schools with a significant population of students of color, and the McDonald's restaurants nearby were dominated by youth of color, brown and black, most too young to drive. In this sense, McDonald's often reflects the same racial segregation that organizes social life in school, as we saw earlier in the cafeteria.

In the case of the Hampton McDonald's, a number of youth who go there reside outside the immediate community and are bused in for school from lower-income areas in the county and thus depended on school transportation to get home.[24] This turned out to be quite relevant since many of the kids came to this McDonald's before practice and games since they could not go home. Again, we can see how schools, by default, serves as feeders to commercial food markets. On game days, there are usually two hours between the end of school and the start of the game, and in this sense, the school calendar and sports seasons and cycles structure the patterns of student participation.[25] At Hampton, there was often a sense of kids killing time either between activities or before having to return home. I remember that on one Friday, a game day, one boy remarked to one of his friends at the tightly crammed table where he sat, "What are we going to do for the next hour and a half for real?" McDonald's and other commercial outlets become way stations, absent adult authority found at home and school. (The football coaches at both Washington and Thurgood coordinated after-school meals for their players in order to provide an alternative to these commercial foods since many players were hungry before games and practice. Likewise, Dan provided meal services after school for Washington athletes.)

I also observed at Chipotle because Chipotle was discussed favorably in almost every interview conducted, especially for its hefty burritos and fresh guacamole. While I visited several Chipotles, I consistently returned to one in particular, which is located just under three miles from a neighboring high school that I refer to as Riley High School. Because of this distance, easy movement between Chipotle and school is all but impossible. Riley High School is a very large secondary school. The population of students is mostly white and Asian, with parents who mostly belong to the educated, professional classes, as do most in the surrounding community, and this is well reflected at Chipotle. Participants are typically Anglo, and to a lesser degree Asian. Access is usually by car. I sometimes watched mothers in minivans drop kids off outside Chipotle.

While students may frequent Chipotle once a week, students return to McDonald's daily. Cost matters, of course, and has consequences for how frequently youth customers return. Unlike McDonald's, which has an expansive dollar menu with various offerings and allows for the purchase of a burger, fries, and a drink for three dollars, a Chipotle meal, which is usually some variation on the "Mission" burrito, when including a drink costs upwards of nine dollars. While I saw instances of kids getting chips and guacamole, which runs about three dollars with water, a burrito and a soft drink were far and away the most popular menu item for these high schoolers.[26]

These financial considerations explain why kids could be found after school day after day at McDonald's, instead of other places, but in the end cost tells only half the story because it doesn't sufficiently account for the collective life of fast-food hotspots. This is the case because, as I have already suggested, participation in the public commercial food realm provides a means to participate in public life. Youth have long seized consumer spaces for their own ends. As many youth scholars have demonstrated, youth's struggles for freedom and independence and claims of cultural authority are often made meaningful in the consumer sphere.[27] Making sense of youth's participation in fast-food hotspots like McDonald's, then, has much to do with youth identity work and friendship networks in public space.

The Collective Life of Fast-Food Hot Spots

In the fall of 2009, I decide to stop in at the McDonald's across the street from Edwards High after school. When I arrive the place is packed. The front entrance is nearly blocked by a wall of boys, black and white. One boy, short and stocky, wearing a trucker's cap with a mop of dirty blonde hair underneath and a face full of acne, stands at the door. He has on a red, oversized t-shirt and skater jeans, wide in the leg and ending a few inches above his high-top sneakers. He boisterously talks to a black kid, also outside. The inside of McDonald's is flooded with kids, most in jeans and hoodies. Earbuds are ubiquitous, as is the black backpack over the black puffer jacket. I come in, get on line, and order a coffee. The line is long, so I stand there for ten minutes, watching kids come in and out and approach each other as they too wait in line. Many kids know each other, and like the Hampton McDonald's, this McDonald's seems like an extension of Edwards High School. The crowd is mostly black and brown with the exception of one full table of white kids and me. I grab a seat and soak in the scene. I spot a girl working quietly on homework—but she is the only one. The kids all seem to be talking, though none are yelling. This is a kid's space. I overhear the white group—comprised of three girls with little trace of make-up and three boys—talk about buying five-dollar apps. Two white boys sit at a taller table. They seem older, maybe seniors, and are chatting as a black girl, dressed in leggings and layered shirt and long faux pearl strands, approaches them, asking, "You save me any?" She sits with them and the three of them talk for the course of my time there. I overhear someone ask, "You got two cents?" but I don't hear the reply. A black boy dressed in what looks like gym clothes—black athletic shorts and a t-shirt—puts his bag and cell phone down and walks toward the counter. He quickly returns and says aloud, though his remark is not directed at any one person, "I just left my phone right here, anyone could have stolen it." He picks up his phone but leaves the other stuff behind as he walks outside to stand with the boy in the red-t-shirt and smoke a cigarette. Several kids are mobile in the scene, moving easily from one table to the next, some appearing to never sit down. The easy mobility and freedom of movement is what is most valued in this setting. This is hardly revelatory given the deeply constrained character of movement in the confines of school hallways, classrooms, and cafeterias. And thus, this space can be understood as a setting where the restraints of movement and the constraints of the body that we associate with school are left at the door.

While McDonald's may belong to a lexicon of "fast food," for these youth there really is nothing fast about it. Unlike in school, time slows, and the standard chunks of time between a ringing bell are cast aside. At McDonald's kids linger, stretching not just dollars but time. The easy movement within the interior space of McDonald's and the contrast to the cafeteria space at school, then, pattern the way youth define and occupy this commercial setting. McDonald's, at least those I observed, is at once an extension of school and a radical departure from it. Students move in and out of the McDonald's, go back to school, and then come back again. There is a literal revolving door of kids—often the very same kids cycling in and out several times over in the course of an hour. Talk of teachers, coaches, and homework dominates their conversations.

On many occasions I arrived to a rousing scene at these McDonald's restaurants, with teens talking loudly, yelling to each other across tables. Their actions exaggerate their sense of claim to the entire McDonald's space. On one afternoon early in the school year at Hampton, I arrived to a bustling scene. The volume of the store increased rapidly as kids filtered in. Two boys floated into the restaurant, heading slowly past the counter toward a collection of six boys; all, with their clean athletic shoes and exercise gear, stood in a loose circle huddled close to the counter. Their mood was one of exuberance—their energy bubbling up and spilling over to those standing in line beside them. The volume of chatter continued to rise and then was pierced by the shrill cry of a girl's voice as she screamed, "Get OUT?" and then collapsed in laughter. "Nooo waaayy!" I spotted out of the corner of my eye a table of three guys. One of them was singing, slightly off-key, as he moved rhythmically in his seat while listening to his iPod, earbuds fastened in his ears. From behind the counter a clerk's voice rang out, barely audible over the din, "Number 4." No one claimed the order, and he yelled out again. His voice was followed by a girl from the crowd who yelled out, and loudly, "Number 4." The bag was claimed.

The boundaries between tables at these McDonald's settings are fluid; there is a continuous refashioning of table arrangements, with moving chairs and the spilling over of bodies onto other tables. Stretching and reworking space, kids colonize areas claimed by others. This could be seen on one occasion at the Hampton McDonald's when a boy standing a few feet from me sat down at my table. With his eyes glancing toward me, he waited for a response. His friend at the booth across from my table interjected, "He's mentally ill," as the other boys at his table chuckled in response. At this, the boy stood, pushed in his chair, and retreated back across some invisible line that separated the few adults present from the kids.

All three of these McDonald's restaurants look, sound, and feel like kids' spaces, a feeling symbolically conveyed through tone and types of talk, movement of bodies, and the reworking of the physical arrangements of the space. I remember on one occasion I arrived to the Hampton McDonald's, took a seat at a table with four chairs, and spotted a group of six boys, all black, with closely trimmed hair, jeans, sneakers, and t-shirts, with "Hampton Football" written on several of them. The tight huddle they held a moment previously dissolved as a few headed to the counter, others slipped into booths, and one turned around and headed back outside. Two boys sat in the booth cater-cornered to me, and the table in front of me had three boys. The space between tables was narrow, such that if one boy stood between two tables, he could be part of both, a fact I observed countless times. There was a tangible sense that tables are not distinct entities.

Importantly, adults do not linger at these McDonald's restaurants after school. As one of the only adults in the space, I was a bit of an aberration, a curious fixture in the scene. Workers, almost all immigrant adults, absorbed in the busy work of food orders, typically remained behind the counter and thus were symbolically cut off from where the action was. The few parents who came in with kids gathered their food quickly and left. I was often struck by the bemused smirks exchanged between lone adults, whose departure was typically swift. On one occasion a man dressed in the uniform of a security guard entered the place and moved toward the counter. He was a very large man and looked quite serious. Many kids took note of his presence, boys in particular, and I heard the sound of "sshhh" from a crammed table of five boys as the room momentarily went silent. They registered his presence but did not alter their action in any significant way as the cacophony of voices returned within seconds. Two other boys blocked the aisle, one leaning on a table. And the security guard had to navigate his way around these kids to reach the counter. He was an interloper. For the sociologist Rick Fantasia, who studied McDonald's in Paris when it first opened, the absence of adult supervision helped to explain the draw of McDonald's for Parisian youth. The counter where food orders are placed separates the adults from the teens. Self-service, a defining feature of the fast-food experience, reduces contact with adults, helping to explain the appeal of fast-food restaurants for young people in particular.[28]

This, of course, can quickly dissolve, however, as adult authority is easily reasserted. On another occasion, a man in his thirties, stout and stocky, in his Hampton athletic shirt and khakis, walked in and with purpose headed to the line. The volume suddenly rose and I heard, "Coach Peters, why you here?"—to which no response was given. I overheard one of the boys say to the others at a table of five, "We're not supposed to be in here, we've got a game." One of the boys said loudly enough for the coach to hear, "I had Subway," suggesting that he might be here, but he had not eaten here. I had no way to verify this claim, and I heard another boy say, "I gotta eat," as he popped another french fry in his mouth. The coach grabbed his bag, turned, and with head down and his voice stern, admonished, "Let's go," as he headed out the door. A few moments passed. "We out," I heard one boy announce, and several tables of boys began their movement up and out, and they headed back to school for the game.

Yet these moments were rare. More common was that these settings functioned as youth cultural scenes where loose and ever-evolving networks of friendship and group boundaries were displayed, tested, and fortified. In the context of relationships, food became especially meaningful since it served as a tie sign, to borrow again from Goffman, publicly linking two people together in some way.

Gifting, Badgering, and Stealing

Kids spend a lot of time in these McDonald's engaged in negotiation with friends around food and money. In this sense, both money and food emerge as symbolic goods. Food is central in the gift economy of youth both inside school and in the commercial realm, and money among teenagers is often defined as a shared resource. American youth carry the obligation to offer gifts as evidence of the strength of friendship ties and also hold an expectation of reciprocity in gift giving, in a way that is much less evident in adult interaction with food in a U.S. context. In other words, while they expect to be the recipient of food gifts, they are aware that they must also bestow them. These reciprocal exchanges, sometimes a subject of dispute, serve as measures of the durability of social ties and are central to the public display of peer and friendship networks, and thus are important to our understanding of youth's engagement with consumer food markets. The consumption of commercial foods exists in a web of spatially contingent social relationships.[29] A Big Mac, for example, can exist within a complex emotional field, with its meaning derived from a "different sphere of exchange"[30] beside the consumer market. As sociologist Eva Illouz explains, "[O]bjects can leave the sphere of consumption and the market and become incorporated in interpersonal relationships."[31] I witnessed this multiple times. I remember on one occasion watching as a girl at the Hampton McDonald's meandered over to a table where five boys were crammed in, leaning over one of the boys and helping herself to a few of his french fries before turning around and heading in the direction of another table. Her wry smile and fleeting action suggested that she was quite delighted with herself for the successful claim she had made on the boy's food. Hers was a public expression of entitlement to transgress a boundary of familiarity bound to food, an object we ultimately ingest. Gender seems especially meaningful in this exchange. Feminine food scripts are narrowly conceived in terms of either the denial of food for the self or the serving of food to others, as philosopher Susan Bordo has observed, and these scripts pattern young women's relationship not only to food but also to young men. That the action was staged before an audience of all boys made it all the more emotionally charged.

To share food in front of another is to engage in a public display of intimate social ties. Adolescent social norms guide this behavior, as we also saw in the cafeteria. Indeed, the sharing of french fries can have as much to do with the emotionally rife position of peers vis-à-vis each other as with its market exchange, if not more so. The offering of a single french fry to one person over another can be taken as a promissory note of future dealings or signal a severing of ties. In this regard food is an "expressive resource" and a means to solidify the boundaries and membership of groups of friends.[32] Consider this exchange shared between friends, observed at the Hampton McDonald's, as illustrative of this point: "Okay, I have two dollars and twelve cents," I heard a boy announce. This had to be enough to buy something because he started to rise in his seat. A conversation ensued about what he should get. Jeff, one of his friends, said, "Get a Big Mac," to which Amanda, another friend and a McDonald's regular, responded, "You don't need a Big Mac." "Yes, you do!" Jeff insisted. (I suspect Jeff was hoping to claim a bite.) "I'm trying to help you," Amanda pleaded. "It has so much fat in it." Eventually their friend got up, got on line, and ordered himself a Big Mac. When he returned to the table to eat, Amanda and Jeff had moved on to a new topic. But the example hints at the influence friends attempt to exercise over the food choice of others as an expression of friendship ties and highlights the publicly negotiated character of these exchanges in youth cultural scenes. Collectively held friendship "feeling norms," as sociologist Donna Eder calls them, structure these exchanges.[33] The expectation that food is to be shared among friends and the obligation to express care and concern for a friend reflect friendship norms commonly shared among adolescents. Just as spouses hold ideas about obligation and entitlement of gifts of time or work, what Arlie Hochschild referred to as "economies of gratitude," so too do friends. These norms become threads that hold these small collectives together. Food, in this sense, represents what sociologist Allison Pugh has called "scrip," which Pugh defines as a set of cultural things, often (though not exclusively) derived from a commercial sphere, that are "tokens of value suddenly fraught with meaning" and that serve as means to communicate "worth of belonging" and make claims of both status and group membership.[34]

Barter, negotiation, and gifting of both money and food serve as cultural resource, a way into youth conversational worlds. They are a means to secure one's place in a group and thus are part of what Pugh refers to as "the fabric of belonging."[35] In this context fast food is as much gift as commodity, an objectification of relational ties. As Dan Miller explains, goods purchased are "used to objectify social relations, a process in which the social life of things is formed through the object life of relationships."[36] On one occasion at the Hampton McDonald's, I observed as two boys sat down with one McDonald's bag. One said to the other, "Don't be smelling my food." The other boy, sitting across from him at the table, remained silent, and seconds later the boy conceded, saying, "I owe you" as he ripped a piece from his chicken sandwich and handed it to his friend. He accepted the offering and promptly gobbled it up, perhaps before the other boy had a chance to change his mind.

Just as food can be an object around which displays of friendship are affirmed and obligations to others met, so too is money, since it enables the purchase of food. While it is the case that entry to McDonald's is usually not contingent upon money, full participation in the cultural scene does depend on having or gaining money to use for the exchange of food. Failed attempts and successful ones to collect dollars and change from others pepper my fieldnotes. McDonald's is a world of cash, where crumpled-up dollars are retrieved from deep within the front pockets of jeans, and the clatter of dimes, nickels, and pennies can be heard as they are pushed across the counter one by one in purchase of a shake or french fries. Virtually all the kids pay with cash.[37] Not once did I see any bill bigger than a five; most were one dollar bills. In this context tender emerges as a central object, serving to demonstrate and solidify in-group and out-group boundaries and belonging.

Sometimes negotiations around the exchange of food and money look less like gifting and more like badgering, and the expectation of reciprocity is cast in doubt. Every once in a while the refusal to offer food as gift devolves into outright stealing. I witnessed routine efforts by young folks to collect money in a piecemeal fashion. One afternoon, as I sat at the Hampton McDonald's, sipping on an iced tea, watching as I scribbled notes, I overheard a boy ask for money. "I don't have anything," he said, and then paused. "Alison, do you have cash with you today?" "Do you have, Patricia—for me today? I just need fifty cents and I'd be in business. Dime? Quarter? How am I going to find fifty cents?" the boy wondered aloud. This continued for a few minutes before he gave up and parked himself in a seat as he longingly watched others eat. In another instance, a slim, bubbly girl approached a guy and gave him a hug. She looked down at a boy at the table sitting alone and said to him, "Do you want to give me a dollar?" He responded, "I'll give you a dollar if you give me a napkin." "Really?" she asked with noted surprise as she turned on her heels and went off in search of a napkin. She returned, handed him the napkin, and said, "Alright, give me the dollar now." But he was unwilling to oblige her, and she turned her back, quickly affecting a pose of indignation.

In some cases, money was an object of playful ridicule. I watched kids throw change at each other on a few occasions and also saw attempts to playfully steal money from each other. These were dramatizations, an opportunity to gain visibility by others in the scene. On one afternoon in the late spring as I observed, my attention was drawn to a girl wearing green shorts who said, "Stop!!!!" A boy remarked, "I know, you ain't laughing," as he grabbed a dollar out of her hand, to which she replied, "Give me back my dollar, I only have two dollars." She was laughing as she said this, and it was clear that this exchange was performative and playful. In other instances, money was given freely with little expectation of reciprocity. It was often taken for granted that money would be apportioned to friends, and this sometimes emerged as a source of conflict, as was also the case with food. I can recall on one rainy afternoon in early October, as I sat watching a boy who for the previous few minutes had been badgering his friend with requests to share his food. Eventually, with a tone of resignation, his friend said, "Get your food." As in this exchange, I witnessed instances of kids caving at requests for money and food. What often began as a "no" to a request for food later became a reluctant "yes," suggesting the force of these norms of exchange and gifting between friends. Kids will buy food for friends if they have money, and often feel obligation to do so as an expression of friendship. But lack of money, for most young people, does seriously restrict their offerings, as the following example reveals. One of the boys yelled to a boy in line, "Get two McChickens, we'll share." This was met without response. The boy did not relent and charged, "I always give you my shit." A few moments later he said, "I hate that shit," to which the other boy responded, "I have two dollars," and pulled them from his pocket as evidence. "What do you want me to do? I can't pay for all of you." Financial constraint punctuates these moments, reminding us of the financially precarious place of youth as consumers. But it also points to an alternate system of value by which young people in collective youth spaces think about money. For young people in these settings, money often is a shared resource, a social thing that objectifes the strength of social bonds. While for parents, money is gifted and shared within the family unit as the objectification of relations of care, for youth, money is an object around which the obligations of friendship and fairness are negotiated. The expectation that money or food be shared was further attenuated by the fact that McDonald's is a public space. It was easy to overhear these encounters, and thus tests of friendship ties were effectively on display. Notably, this did not happen at fast-food establishments that did not transform into youth cultural scenes. I witnessed none of this at Chipotle.

Play and the Collective Life of Hot Spots

These McDonald's restaurants bear the cultural imprint of youth, symbolically communicated through what Erving Goffman, in his micro-sociological perspective, called "small behaviors" and "ordinary human traffic." Kids sit on the backs of chairs with their feet on seats, lean against tables with rear ends resting on a table's edge. Heads lie on table tops and kids lie out across chairs. They eat each other's food and sometimes throw it. Tone and types of talk also serve to claim the space as a youth space. Kids lay claim to space by using their bodies as a resource to locate this scene outside a middle-class adult realm where rules and more formal moral and aesthetic codes rein them in. Ritual burping, choking, and falling off chairs, all related to embarrassments of the body, are used expressively to craft this as a cultural scene organized by the youth sensibility of *spontaneous play*. I remember on one afternoon earlier in the research, observing at the Hampton McDonald's, two boys made their way over to where Jamie, a sophomore, was sitting, her legs stretching across two chairs with her back to the wall. She blurted out before either could say anything to her, "I'm waiting on Amanda, I'm not alone." The bigger of the two boys took a seat, scooching in across from her, as he leaned in to the table with a warm smile on his face. Alison walked in and said loud enough for everyone to hear, "Oh my God! Jamie, you found friends." At this Jamie responded jokingly, with a trace of laughter, "Fuck you." As this exchange demonstrates, tone and types of talk serve to claim the setting as a youth cultural scene, one where adult authority is both absent and the object against which the scene is constructed. Dramatic outbursts and raucous laughter are common. This is bolstered by routine swearing. "I don't give a fuck about you all." "That's fucked up." "Shit." On one afternoon, I watched one boy walk by a table, as he said, "Where's Xavier?" a moment later declaring with much bravado, "You're disgusting!" to his friend. This was followed by one of the few cautionary statements offered to the group: "They're going to kick us out," uttered by a girl. But they didn't. In fact, they never do. The workers take all of this in stride, accepting that the cultural scene was what ensured the kids' return and the guarantee of revenue.

Herein lies a central draw of McDonald's, yards from school but effectively far enough from it to be a space crafted for and shared by youth. It is the emotional charge, a cosmic bubbling up of shared energy, built up over time, that serves to explain why the same young people return to McDonald's several times each week, solidifying their place as regular customers, the scene as a cultural one, and themselves as a distinct group. Emotional energy captured in both the public displays and friendship ties, in food sharing and public outbursts, then, is central to the experience of the setting and the meanings youth generate, helping to explain young people's return to specific commercial food settings. Food is secondary and largely used for relational ends, as we saw in the last section. Sociologist Randall Collins, building upon Goffman's insight, characterized these situations as moments marked by what he terms "emotional entrainment." The physical assembly of the group and the sense of shared emotional energy is often explosive. This emotional energy, or entrainment as Collins calls it, affirms the solidarity of this group of kids and aligns their behavior to the definition of the situation, that is, as a kids' scene ruled by spontaneity, a sense that "anything goes" and that the rules belonging to other spaces and other situations do not apply.

I often watched as an explosive emotional energy washed over the scenes as clusters of kids focused their attention toward the encounter itself and reveled in the moment. I often arrived to a packed McDonald's scene. Moving through the door, I was nearly knocked down by a disharmony of sound. Groups of kids lingered just beyond the door. Forty-plus kids occupied the small McDonald's on any given day, and I navigated the maze-like structure of adolescent bodies, inching my way to get on line. The boundaries between groups were fuzzy—kids shuffled among groups, reconstituting themselves as part of a whole. In this sense, McDonald's is slow food for adolescents, even as it is fast food for adults.[38]

This is not the case at Chipotle. In contrast to McDonald's, at Chipotle the "expressive fabric," to borrow again from Goffman,[39] leaves one feeling as though one is venturing into an adult space where kids are present in large numbers but do not dramatically reorganize the setting's fundamental spirit or assert influence over the situational boundaries, as is the case at McDonald's. While kids return, they certainly do not do so daily, as they do at McDonald's. Little evidence of solidarity among the group as a whole can be found. On one visit to Chipotle, I noticed the noise level beginning to rise and realized that school had ended about twenty minutes earlier. I looked up and watched as a slow trickle of kids came in the front door. Beside me was a table of four boys, who were later joined by a tomboyish-looking girl. They ate heartily as they chit-chatted among themselves. One of the boys had simply bought a small bag of chips. At another table a girl wrapped her hands firmly around her burrito, tilted her head, and dug in. On another visit, I sat down at a table. I scanned the room and noted only two groups appearing to be high school age, the other tables being occupied by adults, a few with young children. The first three girls, all African American, had straightened hair, and one of the girls was dressed in a preppy style with a broad white headband and crisp checkered shorts.

During the entire visit they ate quietly, talking among themselves. By and large, conversations were contained to individual tables at Chipotle. That is, kids used the tables and chairs as they were intended by store management. I witnessed few improprieties or transgressions that served to construct the setting as one defined by spontaneous action and a youth cultural scene, as was demonstrated at McDonald's. These contrasting definitions of space were expressed in countless small gestures. Take, for example, the practice of refilling drink cups. In both places kids helped themselves to "free" refills. In Chipotle, I saw lots of kids quietly refill their cups with soda. I sometimes heard statements like, "I hope I don't get caught." In the three McDonald's restaurants, I witnessed conspicuous attempts to gain refills. On one occasion, I watched as one kid stood at the drink dispenser, filled his cup, drank, and filled it again. His eyes moved quickly around the room, a devilish smile emerging across his face. He seemed to be both trying and not trying to be noticed. His was a public act.

In contrast to Chipotle, at the McDonald's kids lay claim to space by using their bodies as a resource to position this space as belonging outside of a middle-class, adult realm—where formalized aesthetic and moral boundaries rein them in—and instead as a situation crafted through interaction and marked by spontaneity and play.[40] As we saw in the cafeteria, the body is a central resource of spontaneous play in these settings. On one occasion I watched as four girls sat at a table. One playfully slapped the other as they giggled, and one girl kicked the other under the table but playfully, as they took each other's food. The girls were giddy. Suddenly, one girl lost her balance and fell to the floor loudly and flailingly. It was sudden but felt staged. A clamor of loud voices and laughter made it difficult to hear exact words, but the girls found this hysterical. The girl on the floor was laughing at herself somewhat sheepishly as she got up. I witnessed many bodily transgressions at McDonald's (though only a few at Chipotle). Burping and falling off chairs, while embarrassments of the body, are also used expressively to disrupt spaces and their governing interactional norms. While middle-class adult behavioral norms and aesthetics aim to erase traces of the body, thereby placing food in the symbolic realm alone, this is not the case for these youth, who seem to delight in a desacralization of the body through their play.[41]

Youth at the McDonald's capitalize on the body's potential in this re-gard, relishing these moments to disrupt the balance of the situationally appropriate through play. At these three McDonald's settings, kids ac-tively exercise their freedom, unrestrained by adult edicts that rein them in elsewhere. Eviatar Zerubavel argues that a play frame allows for "sym-bolic obliteration of the social order. . . . [P]lay is a perfect vehicle for challenging conventional classificatory schemata."[42] While one might be tempted to interpret these behaviors as oppositional or resistant to adult control, I would caution against doing so, and instead suggest that these behaviors are expressions of the definition of the situation. As Goffman classically wrote, "Not then, men and their moments. Rather moments and their men."[43] By this he meant to suggest that it is the structure and definition of situations that pattern behavior and not the individual par-ticipants themselves.

McDonald's, then, should be considered a quasi-public commercial food space, where groups of youth congregate outside of institutional limits of school and home, that serves as a place of spontaneous play. Jan Nespor has argued, "[K]ids value settings for the possibilities they allow for bodily play and performance."[44] Spontaneous play and action are built up through the interaction and produce a distinct situational spirit that carries tremendous appeal for young people.[45] The cultural logic of these spaces, crafted by youth for youth, is intended to be ap-preciated by youth alone, to mark the distinction between youth and adults, and to provide a map of the boundaries of belonging and friend-ship. Food is taken as an expression of the durability of friendship ties. As teenagers work to craft spaces as belonging to a youth world where a spirit of spontaneity prevails, the boundaries are fluid, ever negotiated, but iterative. By this, I mean to suggest that they depend on a regular public enactment by youth as a collective that is built over time through repetition.

McDonald's, then, provides a stage for a distinct form of play that is tied to the performance and display of a shared identity as youth—a meta-story, if you will, that youth tell to themselves about themselves. This, it turns out, is of primary importance to explaining why youth return to McDonald's daily and visit Chipotle much less often. If we accept the sociological truism that the routine interactions of daily life are fraught with symbolic importance about the social organization, collective life, and membership of groups, then we can see these exchanges as serving interpretive ends through which youth make sense of their world and the collectives to which they belong. The emotionally charged interactions, taken as a whole, constitute McDonald's as a youth cultural scene, where youth provide comment on their own social existence as youth.

Thus, while cheap burgers and salty fries play a role in attracting kids to McDonald's after school, in the end the food tells only half the story because it fails to account for the collective life of McDonald's as a fast-food hot spot and its symbolic structure. Participation in the public commercial food realm provides a means to participate in collective life, to stake a claim to public settings and transform them into cultural scenes. And it is reflexive in that the performance provides a working narrative by youth for youth about what it means to be a youth. McDonald's seems to know this. Public health researchers and policy workers attempting to reduce young people's consumption of fast foods should also recognize the symbolic means and ends youth pursue through McDonald's.[46] Much policy discussion around young people's health, nutrition, and fast-food markets has focused on deceptive marketing, paying much less attention to the collective gains youth draw from their participation in fast-food settings. While a focus on the aggressive and near-ubiquitous marketing of commercial food to youth is important, I think it equally important to ask what youth stand to gain from their engagement with commercial food markets as campaigns to reduce youth's consumption of fast food are adopted and policy is written. Youth have long seized consumer spaces for their own ends. Their struggles for freedom and independence and claims of cultural authority often take dramatic form in the consumer sphere. But it is also a space where youth publicly demonstrate for each other their social identities as youth, providing a narrative for each other as to what youth are supposed to do and what constitutes fun. Herein lies the importance of McDonald's.

Conclusion

Today, food consumption is a principle means through which American youth gain access to a quasi-public commercial realm. Yet a tenuous relationship does remain as youth forge ties in and to commercial food spaces. Their money buys them access, allowing them to linger if they choose; they are an important source of revenue for many fast-food restaurants. At the same time, their presence, especially in large numbers, can generate adult concern about impending trouble of different sorts, in some cases leading to coordinated efforts to remove them from these spaces. As much as they are welcomed by the consumer market for the revenue they provide, youth, especially if black or brown, continue to be seen as a threat to public order. This tension patterns the status of the teen consumer meaningfully but unpredictably, such that one McDonald's might coordinate the timing and availability of its lunch and breakfast menu to correspond with the school lunch period in order to maximize sales, while another McDonald's might close its store at 10:00 p.m., keeping the drive-through window open until well after midnight to prevent teens from occupying its tables, while not foreclosing the store's ability to collect their money. This also has relevance for understanding the after-school rush, the period of time when youth are most likely to congregate in youth groups. For adults, the period between 2:30 and 4:30 in the afternoon is a down period between lunch and dinner. In the world of retail food sales, the lunch rush has ended and the dinner rush has yet to rev up. The after-school rush, then, represents an important revenue stream for many fast-food restaurants, and thus is often welcomed, even if it means forfeiting the space to youth cultural ends, which is precisely what happens at the McDonald's stores where I observed. As a result, youth were rarely policed in these commercial settings.

McDonald's stores are often a close walk to high schools. Their proximity, and their low cost, create the conditions for the production of youth culture that provided significant revenue opportunity for them. It is much easier to buy a friend french fries and a one dollar burger than a seven dollar burrito from Chipotle. Thus Chipotle, while winning on taste (and, as some claim, health) does not provide opportunity for the display of group membership through gift giving and exchange. Nor are the conditions as ripe at Chipotle as they were at the McDonald's stores I observed for collective and playful displays of youth identity work that youth perform ultimately for themselves.

Understanding the meaning and experience of everyday consumption of fast food in commercial settings by youth requires attention to the role and relevance of social-spatial relations of consumption, or what Erving Goffman famously called "situations." I have mapped how the emotional landscape of these situations creates a "condition of heightened intersubjectivity"[47] that provides meaning and motivation for the continued return to McDonald's by these kids.[48] Little attention has been given by scholars to the role of the situation in structuring the way youth consume food and what they consume.[49] To understand why young people return daily to McDonald's, I have drawn attention here to two relevant aspects of the situation—the socio-spatial dimensions of the situation, their links to the expressive behavior; and the resulting emotional charge of spontaneity and play and the display of friendship ties in gift giving, witnessed in commercial food scenes. I have suggested that a useful way to proceed in understanding youth's food consumption is to ask not "what do kids eat?" but "*where* do they eat?" My answer has been, they eat in situations. While young people quickly grow tired of the routine and limited menu at school, they rarely grow tired of the McDonald's menu, which is also narrow in its offering. This is the case because the scene, one marked by spontaneous action, is always changing, so the food doesn't have to.

Youth themselves play an indispensable role in the consumer food event for other youth, directing our attention to the importance of interpersonal relationships and embodied experience structuring youth's relationship to objects (food) and consumer space (fast-food restaurants), but in a way that extends beyond the usual framing of peer influence as "peer pressure," something that is measured in studies examining young people's food choices. It is not so much that young people are choosing to eat french fries because their friends are pressuring them to do so or because their friends fail to suggest healthier alternatives. Instead, it is the case that these food environments are settings for the production of a youth identity and culture and a youth community to which many young people are drawn; they are lovin' it.

Conclusion

Food Futures and Social Change

On February 1, 1960, four black college students sat down at a lunch counter at a Woolworth's in Greensboro, North Carolina, and politely requested lunch. They were refused. When asked to leave, they quietly held their course. Their actions inspired a youth-led movement of civil disobedience centered on equal access to the spheres of public and commercial life. In the years that followed, sit-ins at Woolworth counters throughout the segregated South were staged by youth. In one particularly arresting picture from a sit-in in Jackson, Mississippi, we can see students seated at the counter. They are soaked in coffee and ketchup and covered in sugar. A crowd of young white men, faces full of contempt, stand behind them. In these moments food is transformed into an object to defile and degrade, reminding us again of the symbolic importance food carries.[1] Students were key figures in the civil rights movement, demanding that common dignities be extended to black folks as full citizens. That young people seized commercial settings is not insignificant, as these were after-school hangouts and were central to participation in public life.

Much has changed since those early days of civil protest. Young people move more or less freely in the consumer realm (with some noted exceptions); access to fast food and speedy service, a hallmark of America's modern age, is given for the most part without rebuke. Processed food is inexpensive and readily available, even in our nation's poorest communities. Young people, irrespective of race, represent billions in revenue to food and beverage industries. If overcoming exclusion from the consumer realm is no longer the yardstick of freedom for young people and access is extended more or less to all, what, then, does youth's presence in the consumer realm represent?

Today, in the United States, young people's food lives are totally immersed in the commercial realm; marketers dedicate endless hours to unraveling the secrets of what foods appeal to youth, and in the process, narrow the range of possibilities for young people in terms of identity making, their social relationships with peers and adults, and the way they engage health, transforming their relationship to both public and private spheres of social life. And while youth's food consumption has become a high-priority policy matter as anxiety about childhood obesity, commercial marketing to youth, and a steady diet of cheap, processed foods inside and outside of school grows apace, we know very little about how young people themselves engage the contemporary food landscape, or the meanings that mediate their food consumption. We often talk about young people and food with broad-brush strokes, ignoring the dynamic, sometimes contradictory, and even unexpected ways in which gender, class, race, and place pattern the types of relationships youth develop to food and the meanings they generate about food. Too often we rely on recycled (and often incorrect) ideas about young people's food consumption: masses of girls are trapped in a perpetual state of starvation, lower-income children are the ones who miss out on the family meal, kids refuse to eat fresh, healthy foods in school, children are brainwashed by commercial food markets. In doing so, we elide the central role of social context: the impact of community, school, family, and peer groups, as well the broader historical context of political and economic change and social and cultural transformation, that together shape the variable meaning and engagements with food by youth.

Without question, food is bound up with and shaped by the commercial logics of late capitalism that have meaningfully reorganized daily life at the dawn of the twenty-first century, shaping the systems of value that give meaning to food and our consumption of it. But what does this look like in actual settings where young people eat? This most basic question inspired this project. Part of understanding markets in everyday life means understanding the complex negotiations that occur with them, through them, and in them. Meaning patterns our actions both within and outside the consumer realm, and youth decipher food through cultural categories already in play, many originating from food markets, but many also originating elsewhere. Take, for example, a 2010 drive-through rap for Arby's, made by a teenage boy and his friend. "Wait a sec, wait a sec . . . it's an order for two, I want two roast beef and a beef au jus. I hope I stay in shape and I don't get fat. You know what? Who cares, add a fries with that. A drink, and a shake, and a junior deluxe, wait homey, will that give me acid reflux?" In this case, the commercial market is used as a platform to playfully engage with a contemporary lexicon of health and our current preoccupation with obesity. Whether this is intentional is hardly the point. The fact that fast food is now widely recognized as unhealthy and "bad for you" by well-meaning adults in positions of authority over youth helps to explain this playful engagement. The field of meaning that shapes this type of play is complex and sometimes quite opaque. What is clear is that the more diffuse the meanings, the greater likelihood they will be seized as an object of play by youth.

To answer the question of how young people's food practices and preferences are patterned, other questions must be asked first. How do commercial logics influence (though not determine) youth's meaning making around food? What sort of value does food hold for youth as they move from home to school and commercial realm? How do institutions of family and school respond and adapt to the push and pull of market forces and economic and cultural change? What can food reveal about the changing relationships among daily family life, school agendas, fast-food markets, and young people's relationships to them? To understand why kids go to McDonald's and other commercial places, we have to understand what's going on in school and at home. These questions have guided this inquiry.

Yet these questions also cohere around a much broader set of concerns about the relationship between cultural life and the ongoing production of social inequalities. Excavating the everyday food landscape peopled by youth, I have sought to understand how culture, that is, the shared social meanings and collective social actions that comprise daily life, express, reproduce, and refigure social inequalities as youth move across the institutional spaces of school, family, and commercial realm. Youth's food consumption, more than anything else, is a sphere of cultural meaning—emerging in practice, occurring across different institutional contexts, and patterned by different actors. By this, I mean to suggest that youth food consumption involves more than a set of preferences and behaviors demonstrated by youth. It is a sphere of value that is nearly impossible to separate out from the structuring force of social inequality. To look at food is to look at how social inequalities pattern its consumption. As much as food unifies and fortifies social bonds, it also serves to divide. Youth food consumption is often used to classify and determine group boundaries. Groups of all types are sorted through food. So aware of this fact are food corporations that Pizza Hut, for example, opted to keep their pizza on the à la carte menu rather than as part of the National School Lunch program, to avoid their brand being associated with the poor.[2] Fast foods are classified through evaluative schema and then used to draw symbolic boundaries that tie particular people to particular foods, helping us to communicate the kind of person we are in relation to others, the value and commitments to which we subscribe, and the mental maps we use to divide up and organize our world.[3]

Food consumption is also a central means through which young people constitute themselves as having membership in distinct youth cultures and thus distinguish themselves not only from other age-based groups but also from each other.[4] Most scholars agree that youth consumption is not simply an economic activity but is deeply symbolic in its organization. For many youth today, participating in the consumer food realm is a defining feature of being young. Youth's struggles for freedom and independence and claims of cultural authority are often made meaningful in the consumer sphere.[5] Looking at the time young people spend in fast-food settings following the end of the school day demonstrates how the exchange of food in commercial settings, while serving to knit together groups participating in a collective encounter, also provides opportunity to engage in forms of play whereby youth create a narrative about themselves, for themselves, outside of the institutional confines of school and home where more clearly etched social roles and rules guide them. Through play, food in the commercial realm is decommodified; its importance lies in what it allows in terms of youth identity and the bonds of friendship and peer networks.[6]

The theme of play has run throughout this book. Play is an important element of the way youth engage food for youth cultural ends. We saw how play both enables and constrains the social worlds that youth construct and inhabit, and the central role of food in that play as they ate lunch in their school cafeterias and moved in and out of McDonald's after school. Focusing on play in youth's consumption of fast food casts light on the significance of collective energy, as well as of situation and setting, to collective action in the commercial realm. It is the emotional charge and sense of spontaneous play these scenes promise that draw these kids in, ensuring their continued return. Such a direction highlights the role of identity, emotion, and social bonds in consumer encounters that have relevance for the way scholars and advocates for food policy and behavioral change address young people's food consumption and health.

Aesthetic and moral considerations also come to bear as we contemplate the meaning of food play. In Bourdieu's formulation of class and culture, taste is a system of distinction that serves to reproduce domination and is expressed principally as an exercise of *dislike*. To be sure, children's and teens' gastronomic longings, while often classified as unsophisticated and simple, are also regarded distastefully by large numbers of adults. Young people capitalize on this, relishing moments to gross out parents, teachers, and other supervising adults, to playfully disrupt social boundaries.[7] The types of food play observed in both schools seemed to operate by this very logic, accepted by adults on some level as what Pierre Bourdieu characterized as "youth allowed its fling."[8] Recall some of the "food pranks" observed at Washington, as a type of limited liability play by which youth not only pass the time but also provide comment on the public institutions that house them. Through these forms of play, youth identity and adolescence as a stage in the life-course are made recognizable. In this sense, food play has a generative dimension, helping to create social categories that structure our everyday social reality.

Of course, these forms of play and spontaneous action render invisible the relations of commodity exchange in which youth are engaged, displacing a focus on markets and consumption in favor of a focus on youth themselves. We certainly should not ignore the fact that young people are spending money on food derived from an industrial agricultural complex, that a large chunk of their time is spent in commercial settings, that the market does restratify youth groups, and that there are tangible health outcomes for youth. But it is youth's meaningful engagement that shapes this field of meaning and action.

Food, Anxiety, and the Modern Age

One reason food is so readily seized by youth as an object of play is that it is an object of such anxiety for adults. Recall the playful rap discussed earlier. Adult anxiety inspires youth play. Worry over the perils of excess consumption by young people—whether we are talking about drugs and alcohol, video games, gangsta rap or rock n' roll, or soda and french fries—is nothing new. Certainly this concern can be noted as a nation weighs in on the meaning of youth's food consumption and what often amounts to a reductionist line of reasoning about the corrupting market influence on health outcomes. Today the discourse of childhood obesity is everywhere. Raise the question of children and food in a conversation, and you can bet you will eventually be talking about childhood obesity.

What motivates this public drama? Adolescents (and indeed children) have long played strategic roles in national campaigns in the name of progress and change. Remarking on the emergence of "the adolescent" as a moral category of being at the beginning of the twentieth century, Nancy Lesko argues that "in public spectacles, scientific research, popular ideas of health and disease, and political rhetoric, adolescence became an embodiment of and worry about 'progress' and a site to study, diagnose and enact the modern ideas for personal and social progress."[9] We can see a similar set of concerns at work today. The emergence of childhood obesity as a risk category in the early part of the twenty-first century expresses the shared anxieties and uncertainties of parents, policy officials, and other institutional actors at a time when the demands of work for parents in an increasingly global economy have contributed to a social situation where adolescents' and children's daily routines play out in social spheres largely separated from their parents[10] and when worry intensifies over our ability to care for children and ensure a secure future for them and for us in the face of a public retreat.[11]

The questions of what kids eat and who is feeding them have gained serious ground in both public and policy realms, and rightly so, yet are very difficult to disentangle from our anxieties about the precarious fate of childhood. Childhood is increasingly in flux, triggering another set of important questions: Who is responsible for the care of our children? What role should children, especially those edging toward adulthood, play in public life? How should we make sense of the shifting place of young people in a rapidly changing cultural landscape as they move out from under the yoke of the domestic sphere and into a range of public settings? It is certainly the case that young people's food consumption occurs to an increasing degree outside the home, while their food consumption within the home has grown more precarious; yet, in the face of these meaningful changes in our food lives, we continue to see food, especially food served to children, as a familial good and as an expression of motherly care. With food being cast as belonging to the private realm of domestic life, we remain ambivalent about the public provisioning of food in schools. But in our failure to see food as a public good, we reproduce gender arrangements in the home, consign care to the domestic realm, devalue the caring work that is undertaken in public institutions (mostly by women), and exacerbate class inequalities that could be mitigated by public institutions, such as school.[12] It is in this context that private markets step in, capitalizing on this disconnect and in the process both undermining our ability to envision food as a public responsibility and part of a public and widely accessible system of care, and accelerating our drift toward increasing privatization and devaluation of public goods, leading some schools, such as Washington High School, to divest from a public provisioning system altogether. Our growing distance from the more abstractly conceived collectives long associated with democratic citizenship and the public sphere, as many scholars have opined, has diminished our sense of obligation to others, in the more abstract sense of the term, and in the end erodes our political will to bring into being a just and sustainable food system.[13]

Many have drawn linkages between this decline and the contradictions of this current historical moment. This historical period, often referred to by contemporary intellectuals as late modernity, is a moment marked by "increasing cosmopolitanism, individualization, social and geographic mobility, the expansion of consumer markets,"[14] which has enabled a proliferation and pluralization of lifestyles and a growing acceptance, if not embrace, of divergent ways of life. But, this has also been accompanied by a splintering of groups as a basis of identification and deepening inequality. Whereas group membership and belonging, traditionally conceived, was once rooted in collectives bound by place, our increasingly mobile, frenetic existence wrought by a reshuffling of space and time has left us unanchored, creating a crisis of meaningful being characterized by what British sociologist Anthony Giddens has termed "ontological insecurity" and "existential anxiety."[15] For Giddens, this is a defining feature of modernization. In the absence of a sense of place and the erosion of basic trust and easy membership with which to anchor the self, combined with the proliferation of endless choices in the consumer market, the onus is increasingly on us as individuals to forge more personalized group memberships and to craft a coherent narrative of the self, based on the cultural choices we make. In this broader context, food is reconceived as a moral and cultural choice through which group membership and the self are solidified. In this context food becomes central to moral identity claims. Consider the farmer's market and its growing appeal as a viable alternative to what many recognize as a rationalized, impersonal, and alienating system of consumption and production epitomized in big-box stores (ironically conceived as quintessential nonplaces and cathedrals of consumption all at once). At the same time, growing interest in more localized food production, with its focus on knowing your farmer as a way to know your food source, has emerged as a means to manage the specific forms of food risk arising from modernization (consider the concerns about food contamination in industrial food production).[16]

All around us, we can see shifts in the way we think of food, changes in food markets, the expansion of organic offerings at Wal-Mart, sushi in public schools, fruit smoothies at McDonald's—all unimaginable even a decade ago. In this sense, we are witnessing what sociologist Sam Binkley characterizes as a cultural movement, which he defines as "the intentional, shared efforts of loosely affiliated individuals to affect the way people live and think, through the production and dissemination of culture."[17] Cultural movements emerge as collective projects, Binkley argues, under conditions of disruption, whereby some taken-for-granted aspect of our everyday world is thrust from its place in the background to the foreground, stirring reflection and the emergence of new ways of thinking about "the stuff of culture" that in some cases spur action that allows for meaningful change.[18]

I think we can reasonably situate this cultural movement centered on food in the context of late modernity wherein the privatization of goods and services that formerly held public value, an eroding and embattled safety net connected to entitlement programs, the expansion of the consumer sphere where struggles over ways of life are waged, identities formed, and meaning in life found, and the emergence of a risk consciousness all coalesce, forming an existential terrain characterized by uncertainty. Food promises to fulfill our longing for belonging and to anchor our existence in collectives, resolving the uncertainty that characterizes what lies before us.

And as much as we can see evidence of a cultural movement suggesting wholesale change in our orientation to food, this occurs alongside efforts to reverse federal reforms in school lunch as food companies' lobbying arm and its industry advocates expand their reach and reassert their presence in order to recuperate school food markets by applying pressure to loosen the federal reigns on school nutritional standards and provide opt-out for schools in terms of their compliance with federal standards, with direct impact on young people.[19] No doubt, this is a disappointing set of events for those working to effect meaningful change in our food policy and institutional practice. But it does reflect the sustained struggle over ways of life, the contested value we assign to goods and services, the meaning given to public and private spheres of existence that characterize daily life as we move into a new century.

Food, Family, and School

Continued attention to the structural dimension of markets and the practical activities of youth consumers should also proceed with attention to youth's lives in institutional contexts other than markets. For this study, that has meant paying attention to food consumption in school and family life and the changes therein. Of course, this is not to suggest that markets are somehow magically outside these institutional contexts, but family and school, while shaped by markets, also are bound by their own logics.

The cafeteria, for instance, is a window into the dynamics of school life, revealing the sometimes competing commitments of students, parents, administrators. The high school cafeterias at Thurgood and Washington are spaces where multiple lines of social action collide as different stakeholders exercise their influence. What can we learn from the case of Thurgood and Washington in terms of the aspirations and obligations of schools and their food directors to the students and communities they serve? The cafeteria, in all its complexity, provides us with a deeper appreciation of how schools can be meaningful institutional settings that reproduce inequalities even while working to address them. Recall Brenda's efforts to bring into being a food-provisioning system that was caring and just, in recognition of students. In more ways than one, school lunch, the cafeteria and its food, at Thurgood was seized as a symbolic redress to the many enduring inequalities that beckon just beyond the school door but also assume a life of their own inside the classrooms and hallways of not just Thurgood but many schools across the United States. From them, we learn how inequalities between schools and communities can take shape in the most mundane of activities and practices; the cafeteria is a site of struggle over the meaning of school as a public good.

Food directors must manage the dual demands of student participation and student appeal, and in the process navigate the worlds of parents and community and market influence, while also working to address the dilemmas of unequal schooling. Both school food directors were deeply aware that everyone was watching: school administrators, students, teachers, parents, federal evaluators. Thurgood and Washington, different schools on nearly all counts, sought to create healthy learning environments for their students. Both food directors recognized that the cafeteria and its contents were central to that mission. Both recognized the incredible demands of working parents. "You know families aren't home so the kids rear themselves," Brenda opined, echoing in some sense Dan's remarks: "I think they're just really busy doing their career. Easier to give your kids money, if you have money, to let them go out and buy their own food." Yet, at the same time, observations from Thurgood and Washington reveal that a widening food gap between "the haves" and "have nots" is not simply about improving access to healthy foods for low-income families and their children but also about addressing the scaling up of food expectations and entitlements for higher-income kids, both of which shape young people's relationship to a public food-provisioning system. Kids with resources can much more easily opt out of the National School Lunch Program if they find the food to be unappealing and inferior, as can the schools they attend. Many sociologists who study the connections between culture and the reproduction of social inequality have found that inequalities are structured not by resources alone but through the cultural symbols and meanings by which social practices are deciphered. A distinctly class-based orientation to health informed the food choices at Washington; health concerns were often difficult to disentangle from aesthetic and taste concerns of the professional middle class. Contents in the vending machine, for example, were almost identical to the "foodstuff" found at Trader Joe's and Whole Foods, both part of the upscale food market, where many of their parents shopped. The high level of school involvement of professional, middle-class parents created the impetus for the school to better align their school district's food policy and practice with food practices at home, ultimately resulting in the school district leaving the NSLP. In this way, a distinct set of cultural tastes most often associated with members of the professional middle class played an important role in structuring the way food was understood. At Washington, the food served in the cafeteria was well aligned with the distinct class dispositions of its students. In this specific way, the cafeteria served to solidify a form of cultural consumption that has consequences for class identification and also to enable the school to distinguish itself from an ordinary public school. These class dynamics raise concern about the democratic promise of public schools in upper-income communities.

Different forces, then, were at play in structuring the demands food directors must meet and the constraints they face along the way, reminding us how much class matters in the social organization of life inside public institutions such as school. Yet, for the young people who populate the cafeteria, all of this matters much less than who is sitting with whom. For the sociologist, these two realities are deeply entwined.

Both high school cafeterias bear the cultural imprint of youth, but in different ways. Youth engagement with the space of cafeteria at Thurgood was visibly structured by a set of race and gender relations and ties forged to school as an institution that at once sorts by race and class and attempts to leverage its resources to mitigate social inequalities. For Thurgood, deep polarization within the school, easily visible in the cafeteria in terms of who bought or brought lunch and where students sat and what they did in the thirty minutes they had before returning to classes, structured the space. Collective ethno-racial and gender identities are mapped through spatial relations at Thurgood. While it is certainly the case that friendship networks from the classroom will spill over and pattern who sits with whom in the cafeteria, I also sensed a more ambivalent set of feelings held by a group of middle-class, academically achieving white kids, as they sat at the same two tables, removed from the spirited booths, day in, day out, with calculus book open across the table, eating their lunches brought from home. Their actions read like a collective refusal, an unwillingness to engage a space. The focus on books and academics in a space other students worked diligently to define as anything other than an academic one served symbolically to convey their disinterest in this shared space and perhaps even the racial project of genuine integration to which the school aspired, even if it was not fully realized.

Much like many American high school cafeterias, the cafeteria at Thurgood is racially segmented. But, it is also a space where school administrators work to address and to overcome the achievement and opportunity lag to which some students are subject, to build trust and student buy-in, and to forge ties with students most at risk of dropping out of school. Because the cafeteria functions as a social space, perhaps more than any other space in school, it can be a strategic site where faculty and staff can forge relationships with kids without the burden of academic demands of a classroom.

As much as schools provide a setting to examine food as a public good and its public provisioning, examining family life as its unfolds around food production and consumption provides an opportunity to examine how food is conceived as an intimate object, central to our most durable social bonds. While school food is often regarded with ambivalence and is often the subject of intense scrutiny, food and family are intimately, lovingly, longingly tied.[20]

Yet changes abound in modern family life, affecting the way food is produced and consumed at home. Nowhere can this be seen more strikingly than in the changes to the family meal. Examining food preparation and consumption in families across commercial and home sites as they are narrated by young people, we gain a clearer picture from the perspective of youth of the transformation in the organization of everyday family life on what Arlie Hochschild has termed "the commodity frontier." Dan Cook makes the point that "commercial meanings figure integrally in the tussle around food and eating" for parents and their children. And while parents are selective in their engagement with the commercial food realm, as Cook argues, their engagement is not without significant effort and forethought. This is the case because large-scale economic processes have radically refigured how we eat and what we eat. The demands of work for adult family members, combined with the increasing demand of a full schedule of activities for younger family member, leave families pressed to find time and the will to bring into being the daily family meal that is not heavily reliant on outsourced, processed foods. As someone who relies, at least some of the time, on ready-made processed foods, store-bought cakes, school lunches, flash-frozen vegetables, and already-cooked beans from a can, like many parents, I appreciate the easy access of the modern food market, especially when pressed for time. But I think we need to exercise caution in assuming that the modern food market has made our lives easier, and need to press questions about equal access in food markets and the consequences on families.

Perhaps because of the growing complexity of family life, food's symbolic value as a marker of the durable bonds that define what family is has intensified. Hochschild argues that the commodity frontier has eroded and weakened the emotional supports provided by family. She writes, "[T]he harsher the environment outside the home, the more we yearn for a haven inside the home."[21] This helps to explain why the *collective* act of eating carried tremendous meaning for the young people in this study. Food is deeply connected to care and a sense of belonging. Few young people were content to eat alone, even though lots did. "When I sit down and I'm eating with all of you guys, I feel like it's more like I'm eating a meal. I don't feel like I need to eat later because I feel like it's an actual meal," explained Andrea, a college student, in a focus group. It is the collective act of eating that satiates. Another young woman explained why she likes to eat with others: "[L]ike once I'm done, I'm more satisfied."

Yet, our busy lives create fewer opportunities to eat together, especially for middle-class families struggling to *stay* in the middle class, driving them into the commercial worlds of the drive-through, processed snacks, and ready-made meals. At the same time, for families at the lower economic end, uncertainty, immobility, and deacceleration characterize their daily food routines. It is not surprising that the lower the family income, the greater likelihood of shared meals, according the American Community Survey conducted by the U.S. Census. Poorer families will have fewer resources with which to eat out and will be more likely to center their activities on family, since in the absence of the more diffuse networks professional, middle-class people can access, family networks will sustain them. Without the resources to move easily across geographical spaces or participate in a range of consumer activities, many poor children are consigned to a fate of boredom and are denied the dignity conferred to those children with ample resources to demand it and to claim belonging. Sociologist Allison Pugh in her work on class, childhood, and consumption found that these dignity concerns are highly relevant to the way parents respond to their children's consumer desires.[22] She found that upper-income parents were able to resist, refusing to satisfy their children's every consumer want, though these children lived amid consumer plenty in the form of electronics, clothes, and toys. These resource-rich parents engaged in what she called "symbolic deprivation," easily saying no to children's pleas for a range of consumer items because their children rarely had to confront the "dignity injuries" low-income children face daily. Aware that their children often lacked the status items that ensured cultural belonging, lower-income parents engaged in what Pugh calls "symbolic indulgence." Because disposable income is unpredictable for lower-income parents, on the occasions when they had money, they engaged in what Pugh called "windfall parenting," indulging their child's consumer desires the best they could, aware that the money could soon be absorbed by the round of endless expenses. I would like to propose that this framework can also apply to the consumption of commercial foods. Young people often desire commercial foods as an expression of cultural belonging and membership in youth worlds, while for parents food is an object of care. But as Pugh discovered, class patterns the way this unfolds. Perhaps as we work to address youth longing for commercial foods, we might also think about questions of dignity, belonging, and care. Food gifts in the form of candy, bags of chips, Slurpees, coveted items in youth worlds, can be offered as a symbol of parental love and care, just as the denial of these foods and the offering of organic carrot sticks or Pirate's booty in their place can be a moral declaration of care for other parents. As we craft policy and practice to promote well-being through healthy eating, we should be mindful of these cultural meanings and the structuring influence of social inequality in shaping them.

Creating Food Change

Appreciating the complexity of social forces around food is difficult. As one of my students once asked, "Can't a french fry just be a french fry?" As somebody who genuinely likes french fries, including those from McDonald's, I wish it could. *Fast-Food Kids* maps the contemporary food landscape from where youth are located in their everyday worlds of play and care, as they move from home to school, in and out of commercial settings and back again—where food is part of both gift and commodity exchange. I have worked to attend to the discursive and policy frames that inform our current understanding of youth food consumption, with attention to a moral economy, disparities in well-being that manifest in food access and food consumption, and the trends toward marketization in school and home. An important aim of *Fast-Food Kids* has been to make a case for why *the tools of cultural analysis*, with its attention to narrative, the systems of meaning and value that direct action, dignity, affective ties, symbolic boundaries, status rituals, and play, are important to effective public health policy and school food reforms. We derive meaning from our consumption because consumption is deeply cultural in form. As we consume food, we understand food from cultural categories already in play and craft new meaning as we respond to the circumstances of context. But in making an argument for why cultural analysis is important for policy and practice, I do not want to sidestep what are deeply etched inequalities in the structure of social life. They work together. Other problems are in play: declining wages, an eroding safety net, eroding trust in public institutions, and the growing fragility of families create conditions for demand for inexpensive, overly processed foods offered by the commercial market. For many communities, concerns about obesity and other diet-related health problems are tied to the built environment, not just in terms of the number of grocery stores but also in terms of the extent to which young people and their parents feel safe in their communities to use parks and other green spaces. Historically, redlining and lending practices led to uneven development in cities, giving rise to what we now recognize as ghettos. Financial disinvestments, capital devaluation in the urban core, propelled neighborhoods into deep poverty and with it, declining access to healthy foods. We must also attend to these matters as we understand cultural mediations on food.

Not losing sight of the fact that young people's food consumption belongs to both an economic and a cultural terrain, as well as a moral one, bound up with care, is important. Like play, care was a recurring theme across the chapters. Political scientist Joan Tronto explains the public stakes of caring in a democracy. "Caring is not only about the intimate and daily routines of hands on care. Care also involves the larger structural questions of thinking about which institutions, people and practices should be used to accomplish concrete and real caring tasks."[23] Care should remain a part of public institutions and public discourse and not be consigned to the private sphere alone. One way to anchor a language of care in a public realm is through a language of rights. Tronto asks,

> Are there rights to care? Clearly there are at least three. If we believe that there is good reason to take care seriously as a public value, then we need to make three presumptions to provide such care. First, we need to presume that everyone is entitled to receive adequate care throughout their lives; we can even call this "the right to receive care." Second, there is "a right to care": everyone is entitled to participate in the relationships of care that give meaning to their lives. Third, everyone is entitled to participate in the public process by which judgments are made about how society should ensure these first two premises.[24]

The UN Convention on the Rights of the Child (CRC) recognizes food as an important dimension of the right of care, declaring,

> State parties recognize the right of the child to the enjoyment of the highest attainable standard of health. . . . State parties shall pursue full implementation of this right and, in particular, shall take appropriate measures . . . [t]o combat disease and malnutrition . . . through the provision of adequate nutritious foods . . . [t]o ensure that all segments of society, in particular parents and children, are informed, have access to education and are supported in the use of basic knowledge of child health and nutrition.

While the United States has never officially ratified the Convention on the Rights of the Child, local organizations, movement groups, and nonprofits have seized a human rights framework to advance a more just food system in which youth are important players. The Youth Food Bill of Rights, drafted by the U.S. nonprofit Rooted in Community (RIC) at their youth congress, articulates as a basic right the "right to real food." In their formulation, the obligations and rights to care are fundamental to political action. In the last decade, much greater public awareness and increased policy attention has been given to understanding the relationship between community-based social inequalities and health disparities, galvanizing grassroots efforts to create community change and to advance the claim that food access and food security are justice issues. Evidence abounds of growing grassroots work, rooted in a commitment to care, to fix what many recognize as a broken food system that has resulted in some important community-building interventions to improve food access in poor communities and to increase food consumption of healthy, affordable foods among low-income families and expand green spaces, allowing for greater community participation and solidarity. Food justice movements have gained a lot of traction in addressing health disparities and environmental injustice, helping to shift the way we think about food as a human right.

Schools remain important settings to enact these food reforms. But we rely too heavily on the extraordinary efforts of a few to provide care because appropriate public infrastructure of support is not in place. The football coach at Thurgood, for example, fed his players before games and practice, doing the cooking himself in order to keep their stomachs full and to minimize their reliance on fast-food options. At another school, no such effort was made, and thus athletes ate at McDonald's before practice and games, despite a mandate from the coach that McDonald's was off limits on game day. Food bans like that tend to come up against a libertarian streak, and because they are top down from adults, serve to foreclose the type of meaningful dialogue needed for young people to see why they should pay attention. Parental restrictions, another kind of food ban, especially of snack foods, appear to have negative effects on children's weight gain, suggesting that parents need more guidance in helping their children engage in healthy dietary practice.[25] For many youth, campaigns to reduce the consumption of processed foods look a lot like bans against other items: alcohol, smoking, rap music—items that at different times in the last century have been seized by young people to establish their own youth culture, to gain autonomy and project a distinct youth identity.

Lots of kids embraced the idea of healthy eating. "I can't eat anything with junk food. It makes me feel weird," one higher schooler explained in an interview. Other kids maintain a relatively healthy diet in practice, even if they "never think about health," as another girl remarked. Some young people talked about their parents' perspectives and orientations toward food as being those of a "health nut" or "anti-carb" person, and kids also talked about shifts in their parents' eating spurred by declining health of older family members. Yet young people were often pretty hazy about what is and isn't healthy. As one girl explained, "Too much protein is not good for you." And at a Subway, I listened to a girl order a sandwich, and when asked the type of bread she wanted, she remarked with a tone of uncertainty, "The grain? Whatever the healthy stuff is." When pressed to define "healthy," generally young people recognized that healthy included fruits and vegetables and staying away from fried foods. But many young people harbor ideas that are downright wrong, which is another reason why it is important that young people learn about healthy foods in school, in addition to having access to them.

Toward that end, I would urge moving beyond conventional nutritional education in schools to a focus on *critical food literacy*, which entails a broader curricular project that enables students to engage the wide range of concerns relating to health and diet, environment and sustainability, industrial food production and food origins, well-being, community empowerment, and public space. A critical food literacy program, in contrast to nutritional education, is expansive in scope, builds on school, nonprofits, and community partnerships, and advances a critical pedagogy where learning is student centered. Since young people's struggles for autonomy and claims of cultural authority are often sought in the consumer sphere, critical food literacy is especially important. Food reforms also need to deal with what the cafeteria signifies for kids. If the cafeteria is a reprieve from the assault on students' sense of self, a place to protect from dignity injuries occurring in academic spaces, this will have consequences for how young people respond to food changes implemented in school. What are the broader conceptions of schooling in play? And how do students interpret them? The way they define and understand both the broader context of school and the place of food in it will have substantial influence on their willingness to embrace the changes sought or, alternately, to reject them.

Let me be clear here. I am not suggesting that we not promote healthy eating or work to increase our consumption of vegetables, fruits, and whole grains. I am suggesting that we proceed mindfully in our efforts, attending to the meaning food holds for young people.[26] We also need to be cautious as we respond to alarmist rhetoric around childhood obesity as epidemic. Campaigns to reverse obesity trends among the young in some quarters look more like a condemnation of fat, creating a context wherein overweight kids are the subject of increasing scrutiny. I am suggesting that we focus less myopically on obesity and fat and more on broader conceptions of well-being that are attentive to the contexts that both enable and constrain healthiness.[27]

Yet despite these real concerns, now at the end of this project, I remain ever hopeful because of the good work of networks of people and organizations working toward food justice and a farm-to-school funding stream from USDA for grants for innovative and local efforts and partnerships to improve food access, food literacy, a reskilling of school food workers, and equipment improvements in schools. There is so much hope in food, which is probably another reason why it is receiving the attention it has as a locus of change. But food change is the means, not the end. Interventions in food are in the end unable to transform the very system that leads to such disparities. Instead, efforts of this type attempt fixes to complicated problems whose roots do not in fact lie exclusively in food, its production, distribution, or consumption. Yet, this work remains important in that interventions of this type provide opportunity to productively address health disparities through public dialogue and public action, even if not the systems responsible for them.

Most food justice workers I came to know in the course of this project understood the limits of the change they worked for, but embraced a pragmatic commitment to collective empowerment and incremental change. They sought small gains in the short term, all the while maintaining a vision of collective transformation on a broader scale that was born of the small acts taken together. In this sense, food politics and food change are important means toward other types of change. Lots of people, decidedly apolitical, have become involved in food change, and perhaps this can be a catalyst to greater participation in the public sphere of civil action and civil involvement central to our democratic futures. Recall the students who demanded food service at Woolworth's lunch counters across southern states. My hope is that contemporary youth, like the lunch-counter activists, will be recognized as important social actors in their own food futures and its democratic promise.

METHODS APPENDIX

Ethnography, both in its classical form and in its contemporary iterations, is principally concerned with the constitutive link between
meaning and action. The anthropologist Clifford Geertz argued long
ago that the task of ethnography is interpreting interpretive activity. "It
is through the flow of behavior—or, more precisely, social action—that
cultural forms find articulation."[1] I have proceeded with this understanding of ethnography, attending to how meaning and action operate
on different registers: institutional, interactional/situational, individual.
I have sought to bridge analyses of material and institutional practices
and the interaction order, focusing on the processes of everyday meaning making through which youth construct identity, forge social ties,
construct symbolic boundaries, and engage the work of distinction, as
symbolic social action. To situate meaning and action in a broader field,
I have engaged the work of multi-sited ethnography, with the intended
aim to both situate and extend beyond the specific locale or setting.
George Marcus explains, multi-sited ethnography is an exercise in map-
ping terrain"[2] whereby the ethnographer traces an object across different
sites, identifying the "connections, associations and putative relationships"[3] in an effort to capture both context and the cultural logics of
a particular field of meaning. Examining how food differently figures
across institutional arrangements at home and in school enabled me to
gain greater understanding of a larger story about the private and public
provisioning of food: how the cultural workings of markets shape not
only our food consumption but the social bonds formed through it; the
enduring relevance of class; and the role that emotion, the promise of
play, and relations of care play in how food is deciphered and consumed.

I have also used the tools of "institutional ethnography," a type of
feminist inquiry first initiated by Dorothy E. Smith.[4] Smith's project,
which emerged from a critique of standard sociological research practices, is concerned with explaining how our worlds are socially arranged

by a complex of abstract social processes that remain largely invisible to us as we engage in the mundane activities of everyday life. Smith calls for a *method* of inquiry that emerges from the actual site of social existence, where people live and breathe, arguing that sociological concepts and categories for analysis that originate outside of the everyday world in the end distort more than they explain. Seeing this as central to sociology's role in reproducing power and ruling, institutional ethnography often requires suspending abstract concepts that derive from the textual worlds of sociology and instead privileging a model of analytical induction through which concepts and categories of sociological relevance can emerge from the field. In this same way, *Fast-Food Kids* explicates how a bundle of economic and social relations, as they are concretely organized, informs and constrains young people's food lives, while also coming into being through them. Thus, I am grounded in the local and ongoing relations that constitute young people's everyday worlds, but have proceeded with attention to the relations that originate outside their everyday worlds, recognizing that youth worlds are shaped by historical processes unfolding in economic, social, and political realms, not independent of them.

I began this project with a loose understanding that larger-scale processes were at work, but how they were given form and expression in the sites of investigation remained unclear at the outset. As most ethnographers can attest, the early days in the field are inchoate and often quite opaque. It is in this way that ethnography is an act of faith. We wade in, much is murky, and we begin to collect bits and pieces of this and that, slowly threading together a set of disparate parts, hoping that a coherent whole will eventually take form and that it will help to explain not simply the internal dimensions of the case but also something beyond it. Clifford Geertz wrote that "doing ethnography is like trying to read a manuscript—foreign, faded, full of ellipses, incoherencies, suspicious emendations, and tendentious commentaries, but written not in conventional graphs of sound but in transient examples of shaped behavior."[5]

Methodologically, I also situate this project within critical youth studies. Critical youth studies, interdisciplinary in scope, is informed by a set of methodological commitments that include (a) a sustained concern for and consideration of the complexities of power in the research encounter, (b) a desire to conduct sound ethical research that empowers youth and children, (c) a strong reflexivity that attends to the position of researcher in the field, and (d) recognition of the connection between power and knowledge, and an awareness of the place of social science inquiry in constituting the very groups we study.[6] Youth researchers play a significant role in shaping the social experiences of children and youth, inasmuch as the accounts we provide construct reality as much as they describe it. And thus, some elaboration of how I proceeded with this inquiry is warranted.

A central component of my work, here and elsewhere, has been to deconstruct and denaturalize the categories of adolescence and childhood appearing in popular and scholarly accounts, a commitment also rooted in critical youth studies.[7] In a broad sense, I have been concerned with questions having to do with the sociohistorical processes by which age categories are inhabited. Willard and Austin term this "age formation." Like Omi and Winant's concept of racial formation, a focus on age formation attempts to dislodge adolescence and the adolescent body from the reductive and essentialist framework that presumes that biology is the chief determinant of action, recognizing that like gender and race, adolescence does not inhere in the body. In this sense, there is no essential set of characteristics or disposition that defines adolescence or youth. As stages in the life course, they are profoundly social in nature and often quite varied depending on the range of forces that also structure the experience of being young, among them gender, race, class, ethnicity, region, and place.

Yet, to those who stand outside youth cultural worlds, youth is often treated as a totality, internal contradictions or differences are often ignored, and age is presumed to be the principal determinant patterning behavior. Traces of this were evident as I talked with many adults about youth and food. The expectation often seemed to be that I would discover patterns of eating behavior that were somehow unique to youth that would unlock the means to reverse the downward diet-related health trends that manifest in adulthood. Sure, I did observe some rather curious food choices and habits of eating. But they were hardly uniform.

Informed by the data at hand, I have tried instead to show how youth food consumption is less a discrete activity (e.g., eating) and instead a sphere of meaning populated by a range of institutional actors, with youth among them. I have tried to understand the conceptual worlds from which particular actions spring by excavating the social relations that organize young people's everyday world as they move in and around it.

Observations stand at the center of this inquiry.[8] The collection of empirical materials for this project on youth and food consumption began in 2008 with observing various fast-food outlets. During the initial phase of observation of the fast-food settings in 2008, I visited a number of commercial settings where inexpensive food could be purchased quickly. These included various food outlets not far from public high schools because I was interested to observe in settings where a large number of high school–aged youth could be found. All were located in different suburban enclaves. By early 2009, I had narrowed my sites of observation to allow for deeper understanding of the dynamics of four McDonald's restaurants and one Chipotle. All were postschool destinations (with the exception of the one McDonald's directly across the street from Washington High School). Settings were selected on the basis of their proximity to local high schools because of interest in identifying consumer experience as a group phenomenon, as collective encounter. Two of the McDonald's restaurants were inhabited almost entirely by teens, while at the Chipotle as well as the two additional McDonald's restaurants, adults were also present as customers, which largely determined the scene and my place in it.

In fast-food settings, I sat and observed. To participate more fully in the routines and activities of the settings, I usually ordered something to drink or eat, often a burrito at Chipotle and french fries at McDonald's. On a few occasions I brought my older daughter with me, but most of the time I went solo, a common enough occurrence in fast-food outlets. Much like the kids themselves, I typically stayed forty-five minutes, in some cases an hour. I talked with kids as the occasion organically arose. Often while standing in line, I would comment on the crowd, and this sometimes triggered small talk. But, most of the time I remained a quiet observer. Like the sociologist Erving Goffman, I kept the focus of observation on "ordinary human traffic,"[9] attending to what young people ate but also what they did, what they talked about, with whom they spoke, how they grouped themselves, and how they related to the physical space as a social space. Jottings were openly recorded in a small notebook and in most cases were written up more fully as extended fieldnote entries after I left the field site. They were later coded for emergent themes through the activity of open and focused coding. As is often the case, researchers are typically able to record slices of dialogue in fieldnotes. The use of quotation marks in the recorded observations presented here designates passages stated directly by the participants. To ensure student and school confidentiality, names were withheld.

Kids noted my presence, but only in passing at the two McDonald's restaurants populated primarily by youth, and at the other settings my presence passed virtually unnoticed. The social organization of the space at the two McDonald's settings dominated by teens facilitated an easier engagement with youth in part because there were few clear boundaries that divided the tables. Kids felt free to ask me what I was doing, though the conversation rarely went beyond that. I always explained I was there in my capacity as a researcher trying to understand the food scene and was working on a project about food and young people. While the idea of such a project was taken as "cool," most kids were intent on returning to their social activities, and I moved into the background. Kids rarely stood talking with me for any extended period, and in only one instance did a boy sit down at my table. In the other settings, the boundaries between tables were clearly drawn, and most of the action was confined to individual tables. There was no collective scene that unified the different groups, and thus I was taken as just another customer among the lot. Having a small notebook hardly made me a standout.

Once I had amassed several months of observation, I began the work of initial coding, though I returned repeatedly to my fieldnotes (and later the interview transcripts and written narratives) as I collected new materials, coding and recoding in light of new data and my evolving engagement with scholarly literatures across a number of topical areas, including food and critical nutritional studies, youth studies, sociology of consumption, and cultural sociology. Coding and analysis of empirical materials followed a model of analytical induction.[10] Though researchers do not come to the task of analysis "intellectually empty-handed," thematic content emerged from the process of systematic coding of the data and not in advance of data collection.[11] For sure, the conceptual scaffolding of our disciplines and the stock knowledge that helps us sort and understand our everyday world is always with us in the field, but our research obligation is to adopt a reflexive posture, in an effort of unearth our conceptual baggage and then to bracket it, in the phenomenological sense of the term. This means engaging an active skepticism toward the disciplinary assumptions, categories, and theoretical anchorings thought to explain action as we work through our materials for analysis. It also means paying close attention to our standpoints and how our own social position shapes this standpoint.

The more time I spent observing in fast-food sites after school, the more convinced I became that to understand what was going on in the commercial realm, I would need to better understand school, its meaning, its mechanisms for sorting, and its social structure. These school processes helped organize the fast-food settings. I had already planned to observe in school, since the subject of school food had grown increasingly fraught in public and policy discourse, and thus I set out to identify potential schools and begin the long and uncertain road of gaining entry to them. It took me months and several rounds of review before two schools agreed to allow me to observe. A graduate student, Nicole Hindert, helped to facilitate my access to the first school, and Dan, the food director at Washington, helped to facilitate access to the second.

OBSERVING AT SCHOOL

Observations in schools followed a similar logic as observations in the commercial realm, though in a shorter and more intensive period of observation. Whereas I could easily come and go in the commercial realm and did so over several years, this is rarely afforded to researchers in schools. I spent two months in spring of 2010 observing in the cafeteria of Washington High School. I usually observed four lunches during each visit and typically visited three or four times a week. In fall 2010, I observed Thurgood High School over a three-month period. Again, I observed four lunch periods each visit and usually visited the school twice weekly. At both schools I jotted notes on a white piece of folded paper as kids moved through the lunch lines, buying their lunch, finding a place to sit, eating lunch, and sometimes throwing portions of it away. During lunch I walked the room, listening to groups of kids talk and eat. And I sometimes bought lunch, usually during the last lunch period of the day. I regularly spoke to school administrators, teachers, and lunchroom staff, more than I talked with students, for reasons I discuss later. Toward the end of my observations, I interviewed the schools' food directors to gain a sense of the role of different institutional actors in the structure and form of the cafeteria, and the larger arrangements organizing the space.

I admit that on my first visits I was struck by the narrow and stereotypical conceptions of cafeterias I had formed in advance of my observing, despite my having already spent considerable time observing in high school settings. I very quickly realized that my perception of the cafeteria had been funneled through a lens of popular culture and teen movies where food fights, rowdy eating contests, and juvenile pranks were an indelible part of the scene. While I certainly saw some of this at Thurgood, at Washington, the school I first observed, I faced a quieted scene—a stark contrast, disrupting my expectations of what I would find. This disruption proved most useful as I proceeded with data collection because it compelled me to make visible my own frames of understanding.

I did, however, quickly adjust to the world around me, settling into the scene easily. Both cafeterias I enjoyed returning to each morning. I welcomed the normal round of small talk as I had become a regular face, for a short time a fixture of the scene. I remember one boy from Thurgood who was developmentally disabled stopping beside me each day and giving me a quick hug before hopping onto one of the long lunch lines.

As much as I enjoyed being in these dynamic cafeteria spaces, I found it difficult to watch some kids sit alone. Some buried themselves in a book, a few genuinely didn't really seem to care; unphased, they were successful in projecting an air of indifference, yet others were so acutely self-conscious, it was difficult to miss. For those sitting alone, I watched as their eyes shifted around the room, aware of the public visibility of their alone status. "Will anyone take notice?" I imagined each asking himself or herself. I remember on one occasion at Washington, standing at lunch as my eyes met the eyes of a boy engulfed by a large, empty table. I smiled, and quickly looked away, pretending not to notice. Much in line with Goffman's dramaturgical schema of defensive practices, I engaged with what he famously called "tact-regarding tact" as I projected an active, civil inattention to his alone status in an effort to preserve, as Goffman would characterize it, his "ceremonial self," recognizing that sitting alone is indeed a breech in the social organization of the cafeteria space.[12] It is in this sense that my ordinary obligations to follow the interactional norms of public life sometimes made it difficult to be a researcher.

And as difficult as it was to see signs of adolescent loneliness, I also found it very difficult to bear witness to poverty, visible in small ways in the passing activity of lunch, especially at Thurgood. As each kid punched his or her pin numbers, revealing on the computer screen for anyone paying attention (few were) the amount the child was being charged for lunch, I could glean who qualified for free lunch, aware that the kids who paid nothing were either poor or part of the swelling numbers of children who are near poor. It is difficult to see kids who live without.

Kids often watched me watching them. I knew they were curious about my presence. In the course of this project I became acutely aware of my age, how much it shapes not simply how kids relate to me but also how I relate to them. I turned forty during this project, moved into my midcareer, and watched the distance between me and the kids I have studied for almost twenty years grow bigger. I have often wondered in the last few years if I might eventually "age out" of studying youth. With each passing year, I find it more difficult to break through and into a circle of kids, to build an easy rapport that erases age distinctions, and to distance myself from the parental role through which they increasingly see me and I see myself. I was in my midtwenties when I first began conducting ethnographic research with young people. Twenty years ago, I found it much easier to simply hang out and on some fundamental level gain acceptance as something other than an adult. I passed much more easily as a "near teen," and because I was in my midtwenties, when I first began studying young people, I often was bestowed a coveted status as a newly transitioned adult, and thus held more cachet.

Officially a "ma'am" to most kids, I am now just your run-of-the-mill grown-up, which conferred on me, instead of cachet, some sort of teacherly authority by virtue of my being an adult. This has triggered a noticeable shift in their behavior. But this teacherly authority has also meant that I am sought out for help. On one occasion at Thurgood, a boy approached me, frantically calling out to me, "I need my table," as he grabbed himself, and then said it again. I realized that he was developmentally disabled. Since I was without any real decision-making authority, I didn't know what to do, was not sure who he was, and for a quick second thought he was joking with me, that is, until a group of boys told me that he could sit over there, pointing to a table not far from theirs, and the boy promptly turned and took a seat.

Some kids took me for staff. For example, one boy at Washington, as he exited the lunch line with a milk in hand, was quick to tell me he forgot his milk, clearly worried I might accuse him of stealing. On another occasion a boy at Thurgood asked me whether he could get into college with a GED. I told him about the state university where I taught and about community college and encouraged him to seek out a guidance counselor as he nodded along. However, by the end of our conversation I remained unsure whether he would take my advice.

All of this is a well-traveled road for youth ethnographers. Access isn't easy, and building rapport takes time; genuine trust is hard to come by. As Joe Foley wrote nearly two decades ago, we are often taken as spies. Access to kids is constrained not only by our adult status but also by institutional controls, especially in a contemporary climate where children and youth are thought to be endlessly at risk. My research was no exception, and thus, the broader field of constraint in which research with young people unfolds was highly relevant to the types of rapport I was able to build, the relations I could forge, and the questions I could ask. The circumstance of my talking with youth in the field was such that conversation arising organically was permitted, but I was not allowed to approach the kids during observation without parental consent. The issue of parental consent, a bulwark of child protection in research, is a major obstacle for the ethnographer in school settings. Schools, because they increasingly operate under a microscope, subject to endless regulations, often adopt very strict policies on access. Schools increasingly have review boards of their own to evaluate research proposals, often denying access outright. Schools have adopted official policies on who can gain entry (Graduate-level students are barred from studying schools in particular districts by virtue of their student status.) and have placed significant limits on the types of interactions researchers are allowed to engage in. All of this makes sense, of course, in a context of intensifying school accountability. Researchers are often perceived to be risky for schools. But this, combined with university gatekeeping in the form of institutional review boards for research involving human subjects, makes the work of ethnography with youth in institutional settings an increasingly imperiled proposition.

Gatekeepers at the human subjects review board at my university during the period of data collection were very strict in their interpretation of the federal guidelines on research involving human subjects, some even obstructionist in their many demands for permissions and consent at various institutional levels. Many university IRBs, fearing an outside audit, too narrowly comply with the federal common rule involving vulnerable populations such as children, thereby creating enormously difficult conditions for social scientists attempting to conduct qualitative research. At my university, the situation was compromised enough that an ad hoc faculty committee of which I was a part convened and was successful in pushing for an inquiry at the university level. This ultimately led to an external review, which identified significant overreach on the part of the IRB office. The outcome was a retraining and reorganization of the office to ensure compliance with federal guidelines and ward against mission creep.

The constraints in place prior to the review, however, had profound implications for this project. Unlike data collection for the project on the high school prom conducted between 1996 and 1998, where I had easy access to kids and spoke with them freely inside and outside school, I was often constrained in my interaction with them, especially in school. As a result, my primary contacts and informants were teachers, administrators, food service workers, and security, all adults with varying presence in the cafeteria. Adults became a much more significant part of the project than I had originally intended because of easy access to them, with obvious consequences for the analysis itself. These constraints also meant I relied heavily on the interviews for cross-checks of the observational data since I had fewer opportunities to do so in the field.

It is in this context that I also found I preemptively censored myself in my contact with youth, foreclosing prolonged conversations for fear I might lose access. I can recall on one occasion as I walked around during lunch at Thurgood, a boy asked me if I was a teacher. I told him and his friends I was writing a book on young people and food. "For real?" he asked, and the three started to laugh. "Well, my name is Lashawn.

Make sure you put that in the book. His name is Hot Sauce," he said, pointing to a larger boy across the table, and the three laughed and the boy called Hot Sauce pleaded that that was not his name. I laughed but made sure not to linger too long, fearing I might get in trouble.

These constraints are not likely to loosen anytime soon and will continue to have consequence for the way we do ethnography. They provide real impetus for multimethod studies since what we can learn from observation alone is impeded and demands various cross-checks to confirm our interpretive judgments.

THE ADULTS IN YOUTH RESEARCH

School officials, though willing to allow me to come to their school, took great care to shape my perception of their students and their school, engaging in a form of what Goffman aptly termed "facework." Vice Principal Edwards spent a significant amount of time talking to me. I was often struck by his level of engagement with me and willingness to offer information about the school, and some of its problems, which in the end I concluded was a way to show me that they are aware of their shortcomings. I also found this at Washington, where the principal on my very first day immediately addressed the two large flat screen televisions in the cafeteria, remarking that they were the "bane of his existence," that they had been a gift from the graduating class, that there was supposed to be a continuous news feed, but that the commercials were a problem, especially those marketing alcohol, which we had both watched only a few minutes before he came over to greet me. On another occasion, early on in observing at Thurgood, another vice principal approached me, asking if I was a parent. I explained my purpose, and his interest was piqued, but he was interrupted by a group of boys behind him who were talking among themselves rather loudly. I did not hear what they said, but he did and admonished them. "Gentlemen, we have a researcher here from George Mason. Is this what we want her to think of us?"

Some adults in the school settings also assumed I was guided by a particular food agenda. Even though I had been purposely vague as to my purpose, most assumed I was evaluating the school's healthy offerings. On one occasion as I walked back into the cafeteria line, one of the cafeteria workers commented to me, "See, Dan is two years ahead of Michelle." He was referring to Michelle Obama's health challenge and the launch of her Let's Move campaign and added with a chuckle, "Now you don't see any overweight kids here."

The "lunch ladies," a group who held the least amount of formal power and authority in school, were very standoffish initially. After all, this was their turf and I an interloper, observing at a time when food service workers have faced increasing scrutiny. I can recall on my first visit to Washington heading back to the kitchen, being met by a table of workers who ushered me very quickly back into the lunchroom, virtually shooing me away. That first week, I was barely tolerated. But I made a point of aligning myself symbolically with them, helping them to sort chairs and clean tables between lunches. Soon, I was welcomed and became the recipient of their small gestures of kindness. On one occasion I was bought lunch—"it's on us today," one of the older ladies told me as she punched in my lunch items. Later, as I interviewed Dan, the same lady brought in a bottle of water for me and for him as she bid us good-bye for the day. At Thurgood, after I had e-mailed Brenda soon after I began observing to compliment her on the lunch I had eaten that day, I was recognized by one of the cafeteria ladies and thanked for the e-mail. (And I wasn't just being nice. At both schools I ate the food regularly, and most of the time it exceeded my expectations of school food.) But as much as the lunch ladies had grown increasingly warm toward me, they did want to know how long I was planning to stay. They often asked if I was "done yet."

Adults also assumed I held a clear set of convictions about food, assuming I was pro-health, pro-organic, pro-vegetable, which in the course of this research I actually became. That I am slender no doubt contributed to the impression that I am someone who cares about food and health. But I often bought french fries at McDonald's too. Sure, they were a prop to blend into the scene, but like the kids, I also relished the salty goodness of deep fried potato. I did limit how often I ate the french fries, mindful that weekly salty french fries were not the best health choice.

I remember on one occasion, one of the Washington teachers I spoke to frequently during lunch remarked as he approached me, "You'd be proud," holding up the bag of organic lunch he had just bought down the street. He showed me the alkaline water he had just paid three dollars for as he chuckled about the seeming absurdity of paying that much for water, a public good (though increasingly privatized with the expansion of the bottled water market). He laughed again, leaned in, and through the corner of his mouth confided that he had spent eighteen dollars for the lunch. My eyes widened, and I agreed that that was a lot. After a minute or so, he then asked me if I had read Michael Pollen's *Omnivore's Dilemma*, a searing critique of industrial agriculture that, though it was not without criticism by food scholars and food movement actors, helped to launch a popular food movement. I had not yet read the book, though it sat on my bookshelf at home. And I told him so in part to counter the perception that I was an organic-eating, health-conscious foodie. On another occasion as I sat eating lunch, Joe, who worked lunch security, came over and sat down with his lunch. A few minutes later the same teacher sat down with us. He chatted about the lunch, saying he had hoped the school year would end with a big bang but instead we got this. He was referring to the grilled cheese Joe and I were both eating. Joe quipped, "What are you talking about? I love grilled cheese." We chuckled and I said the potatoes could use some salt—which was entirely true, but I also was aware that I was working to project a particular self, making sure I was not taken as a die-hard "health nut." Though I am still not a die-hard health nut, it is also true that this research fundamentally changed my relationship to food, cooking, health, and the environment.

INTERVIEWS AND FOCUS GROUPS

My time spent in the field was supplemented with interviews and focus groups. The interviews assumed an enormously important role for cross-checks of the observational data, enabling me to verify, round out, and expand interpretive understanding that was emerging from time spent in the field. Interview and focus group participants were recruited through snowball and convenience sampling, with the explicit purpose of developing a racially and economically diverse pool of respondents. Fifty-six interview and focus group participants were recruited, not with the intended purpose of building a representative sample of youth but to *sample for range*, enabling me to broaden and differentiate within the cases.[13]

A range of income groups was represented among interview participants. Of the young people interviewed, the majority were from middle-class and working-class families, a smaller portion (fifteen) of those interviewed had parents who were part of the professional middle class or the upper-middle class, and a few belonged to the near poor. As is often the case, I was unable to determine the socioeconomic position of a few participants. As a number of scholars have noted, assessing class location is complicated. Most of us have multiple class ties; there is not always a tidy correspondence among income, education, and occupation.[14] To compensate, I also listened for cues about distinct types of cultural capital that might reveal class membership and relied on cultural markers to designate class position: their consumption, their educational histories, their schools' resources, and their family, neighborhood, and community lives. Food is fundamentally arranged by class.

In addition to building a diverse sample in terms of class and race, I also paid attention to immigrant status, family form, type of school attended, and age. I decided to interview 15–18- and 19–23-year-olds because both groups, though different in some important respects, share similar life circumstances. At other periods in history, 15–18-year-olds and 19–23-year-olds belonged to two different stages in the life course. While 19–23-year-olds were once squarely within adulthood, this cannot be said with as much certainty today. Like most 15–18-year-olds, many 19–23-year-olds live at home, or in dorms if they attend college (which gives them a quasi-autonomous status) and have limited financial resources, and adult responsibilities such as food provisioning are typically in the hands of others. While both groups tend to rely on varied forms of adult support, the daily routine of 19–23-year-olds tends to be more autonomous, with more time spent away from home, thus having consequence for their food consumption.

I was able to conduct interviews with a small collection of young people from both Washington and Thurgood, though the broader base of participants attended other schools in the area. Two graduate students, Caroline Pendry and Nicole Hindert, assisted with the collection of interviews and focus groups. Together they conducted half of the interviews and focus groups and transcribed all the interview and focus group materials. I completed all the coding of the interview materials independently.

The bulk of the interviews were group interviews. I generally found the group interviews to be a much richer source of data than the individual interviews. The dialogue and exchange among participants was incredibly dynamic. Participants built from each other's remarks, responding to each other, as well as to the interview questions. All group interviews were comprised of friends or family members. In total, we conducted twelve focus group interviews (with two to six participants for each focus group) and ten individual interviews with young men and young women between fifteen and twenty-three years of age. All interviews were conducted in northern Virginia. Forty-one of the participants were female, fifteen male. Eleven identified as being from immigrant families. Thirty-six were Anglo, five identified as black, five as Asian, eleven as Latino, and seven as Middle Eastern. Eight identified as biracial or bicultural. Twenty-nine of the participants were in high school, twenty-one were attending four-year college, five were in community college, and one had completed high school but was not attending school at the time of the interview.

All of the interviews (which were taped and later transcribed) were largely semistructured with open-ended questions and lasted between one and two hours. Principles of theoretical sampling guided interview procedures, which means that the questions asked changed as different concerns emerged. All the interviews explored questions relating to food consumption at home and school, eating out, favorite foods, and least favorite foods. Questions guided participants to talk about food in the context of everyday life, their daily routines, and the rituals and routines of friends and family members. I asked participants to talk about food provisioning at home, who cooked, what they ate, and with whom they ate it. Participants talked about their memories of food in both childhood and the present day and were asked to think about how they imagined food preparation in the future. Participants were also asked to remark on food in school, whether they brought lunch from home or bought lunch, and what they ate after school. These questions enabled me to situate food consumption in broader repertoires of meaning and action as they unfolded in different institutional arrangements.

In addition to interviews with young people, I conducted interviews with adults who worked within the current food system. In addition to Brenda and Dan, the two school food directors, I interviewed five community organizers who identified as community, food, or health activists or organizers. In 2010, I had begun to develop ties with community health activists working in Ward 7 and Ward 8 in Washington, D.C., and northern Virginia. These wards have the highest concentration of poverty in the city and grapple with a bevy of problems relating to food insecurity and access to healthy foods. D.C. Hunger Solutions reports that Wards 7 and 8 have the city's highest obesity rates and are home to large "food deserts." But they are also settings of grassroots work. In the course of this project, I attended some of the events sponsored by different grassroots organizations working in Wards 7 and 8, including an all-day summit on childhood obesity attended by different community health workers—social workers, public health researchers, nurses, and nutritionists; a community wellness fair in a local park; and a volunteer effort to help build a playground for one of the low-income co-ops in Ward 7 after I had been invited by a nonprofit director I had interviewed. I was able to tap a network of adults deeply committed to creating food change. A large number of these adults were women, and many of them were of color, and thus the work is patterned by gender, class, and race. I was able to interview a handful of them. After an interview with a director of a small community nonprofit focused on wellness, the director took me on a tour of a chain grocery store that had recently opened in the neighborhood where she worked. The store was welcomed by community activists and community members since access to healthy, affordable food was severely constrained.[15]

Accessing the network of adults working to change the food system led to my being asked to serve as program evaluator for one nonprofit. I spent 2012 observing, several times weekly, the activities of the D.C. Farm to School network and the Arcadia Center for Sustainable Food and Agriculture (the D.C. Farm to School network at the time operated within Arcadia), groups working to implement food reforms in Washington, D.C.'s public schools, to increase school children's consumption of fruits and vegetables and knowledge of food origins, and to improve access to healthy, locally sourced fruits and vegetables for families in settings where the concentration of poverty is high and access to healthy, minimally processed food, low.[16] Though the data collected for this group does not appear in this book, it did help to provide a broader context for understanding the changing food landscape and the different movement actors pushing for positive change. My work with this organization provided opportunity to observe a focus group of eight upper-income mothers who lived in the school district where Thurgood is located, but the focus group was not audio-recorded or transcribed.

As a sociologist, I strive to practice a rigorous and honest ethnography that connects evidence and warrant, is rich in interpretive nuance, promises empathetic understanding, and spurs reasoned criticism of existing institutional arrangements. In the end, I hope I have stayed true to those commitments and provided an ethnography reflective of that pledge.

NOTES

PREFACE

1 "Fast-food Facts," 2013, Yale's RUDD Center for Food Policy and Obesity, http://www.fastfoodmarketing.org.

2 "Fast-food Facts," 2013, Yale's RUDD Center for Food Policy and Obesity, *http://www.fastfoodmarketing.org.*

INTRODUCTION

1 Though with exceptions, youth workers can be found in fast-food restaurants and other food retail settings, including Starbucks and many restaurants with table service. Immigrants represent about 25 percent of the total population in the several counties and congressional districts in the area where the research was conducted, though about 40 percent hold college degrees and thus would not be candidates for fast-food service work. Depending on the congressional district, between 70 and 80 percent of foreign born identify as Asian or Hispanic, with between 10 and 15 percent from Africa and less than 10 percent European.

When I began this project I had expected that youth as commercial food service workers would figure more prominently in it, and thus focused on both the consumption and the serving of commercial foods by youth. But when I began to observe in various commercial food settings, there were very few teenagers working behind counters, though I did observe young people, mostly of color, in their twenties behind many food counters. For a nice discussion of youth work see Besen-Cassino's *Consuming Work* (2014), which explores a range of considerations relating to the subject of youth work. Besen-Cassino found that upper-income youth, not lower-income youth, are the most likely to be employed in the United States. These youth workers largely sought employment for social reasons, not economic ones, and rarely worked in traditional fast-food restaurants. She distinguishes between student employment, a largely American phenomenon, and nonstudent workers and the relevance of class. Interview and ethnographic material cast light on the class logics shaping middle-class youth's orientation to work and the relative advantage they encounter in hiring. These youth sort jobs into a scale of value; within the secondary labor market of "bad jobs," there are tiers, with low-status fast-food work and the coveted jobs they claim, which carry high status and significant brand recognition. Class provides distinct advantage in the more desired service jobs since these both depend on and reward aesthetic labor, a type of labor homologous to a set of upper-middle-class dispositions and resources. In contrast, low-income youth, with neither the right zip code nor the aesthetic resources readily available to upper-income kids, are essentially barred from the labor market, excluded from even the most menial, low-status jobs. Examining how race and income pattern unemployment rates, Besen-Cassino found that employment rates, not wages, explain racial inequality in the youth labor market.

2 Sociologist Randall Collins's (2004) conception of interactional ritual to interpret this consumer moment is useful. (1) Bodily copresence and focused attention, (2) emotional energy and shared mood, and (3) membership symbols allowing for the sense of group solidarity, in Collins's formulation, are key resources that transform our most ordinary encounters into rituals. All are present in this moment, serving to rework the definitional boundaries that define this situation as something more than simply consuming ice cream. The sort of ritual play they engage is, of course, gendered, bound up with the adolescent girl body as moral object and the expectation and obligation of ritual care it is due in public by actors and audience.

3 Anthropologist Mimi Nichter (2000) regards this type of "fat talk" as speech performance, which she defines as "a public presentation of responsibility and concern for appearance" (51). This type of talk, Nichter suggests, provides freedom for girls, preempting scrutiny from other girls, and serves a rapport-building function. This is perhaps an inversion of Joan Jacobs Brumberg's (1997) very insightful arguments in "Appetite as Voice," which demonstrate how adolescent girls in the Victorian era used food refusal as a means to exercise influence and control over their worlds, and to manage sexual and moral meaning bound up with the female body. See Brumberg's *Fasting Girls*.

4 We might also think about this observation and others like it as signaling what Angela McRobbie (1993) called "a dramatic unfixing" in terms of femininity as moral category. The commercial realm, where competing frames of femininity exist beside each other, has long been an arena of opening up and closing down gender possibilities (see also Harris, 2004; McRobbie, 1993; Nayak and Kehily, 2008).

5 Nichter (2000) defines fat talk as "a public presentation of responsibility and concern for appearance" (51).

6 These contests often serve to demonstrate one's masculine chops and knit together through collective mockery all-male groups of friends.

7 See, for example, Eviatar Zerubavel's (1991) *Fine Line: Making Distinctions in Everyday Life*.

8 2013.

9 Guthman, 2011; Patel, 2007.

10 1973. See also, for example, Sydney Mintz's (1986) seminal *Sweetness and Power: The Place of Sugar in Modern History*.

11 2001.

12 There has been substantial debate over the nature and meaning of the gift, the principles of gift exchange, and gift economy within the discipline of anthropology, beginning with Mauss and Malinowksi, which have centered on questions of reciprocity, presentation, and alienability. See Chris Gregory (2015), *Gifts and Commodities.*

13 1986: 6.

14 Bourdieu, 1984; Johnston and Bauman 2007, 2015.

15 Eberstadt, 2009.

16 Brumberg, 1988; Bordo, 1993; DeVault, 1991; Lupton, 1996; Wilk, 2008.

17 See Watson and Caldwell, 2005.

18 Lobstein, Baur, and Uauy, 2004.

19 See "Childhood Obesity," Robert Wood Johnson Foundation, http://www.rwjf.org (downloaded Jan. 2, 2014).

20 See "Childhood Obesity Facts," Centers for Disease Control, http://www.cdc.gov (downloaded Jan. 2, 2014).

21 See "Declining Childhood Obesity Rates: Where Are We Seeing Signs of Progress?" Robert Wood Johnson Foundation, http://www.rwjf (downloaded July 25, 2016).

22 1988.

23 Boero and Pascoe, 2012.

24 Johnston and Cairns (2015) also recognized a similar pattern of talk among highly educated adult women, what they refer to as the "do" diet, as an expression of embodied neoliberalism.

25 Bourdieu (1984) discusses how men's participation in food contests, where large amounts of food is consumed in short order, is an engagement with masculinity.

26 See, for example, Besen-Cassino's (2014) investigation of contemporary youth labor.

27 See Guthman, 2011; Lupton, 1994; Mintz, 1986; Nestle, 2002. Important exceptions include Janet Poppendieck's (2010) work on the political and economic organization of school cafeterias, Susan Levine's (2008) history of the National School Lunch Program, Salazar's (2007) work on school cafeterias and ethnic identity construction, Taylor's (2011) and Boero's (2009, 2012) work on childhood obesity, and Fantasia's (1995) and Bugge's (2011) research on youth and commercial food settings.

28 See Miller and Deutsch, 2009; Belasco, 2008; Watson and Caldwell, 2005.

29 In the language of phenomenological sociology, we can think of these as typifications. See Berger and Luckman, 1966.

30 Douglas, 1966; Zelizer, 1985.

31 Cook, 2004: 9.

32 What the Dutch philosopher Rick Dolphijn (2004) has termed "foodscapes," those "immanent structures that are always in the process of change," shaping how we live our lives with food (2004: 8).

33 See Boero, 2009.

34 See "Retired Military Leaders Say This Generation Is "Too Fat to Fight," *CBS News*, Jan. 2, 2014, http://www.cbsnews.com.

35 Bourdieu, 1984: 180.

36 Greenhalgh, 2015.

37 See for example Metzl and Kirkland, 2010.

38 Metzl and Kirkland, 2010: 6.

39 Biltekoff, 2013: 3.

40 Biltekoff, 2013: 9.

41 See Bauman, 2000; Giddens, 1991: Harvey, 2007; Metzl and Kirkland, 2010.

42 2013.

43 Metzl and Kirkland, 2010: 1–2.

44 See "Obese Child Taken from Parent's Home," *New York Daily News*, Nov. 27, 2011, http://www.nydailynews.com.

45 See Boero, 2012.

46 Guthman, 2009: 1113. Antibullying legislation in school tends to omit concern for obesity. See Greenhalgh, 2012 for a discussion of bio-bullying.

47 Statistics, objects of science, have long played a leading role in the crafting of a public problem, because they help to confer legitimacy to it. Think about how often we hear about the rising rate of obesity, the number of Americans registered now as overweight. I even cited them myself in the book's introduction. This is the case because statistics are important in mounting a claim for action or change. But statistics, as they move into the bureaucratic realms of government office and various nonprofit organizations, can take on a reified form, whereby the numbers assume a sort of life of their own. Thus, we need to be cautious in our use of statistics in claims making. Statistics, like all things, arise in the context of meaning, definition, and interpretation. See Gusfield, 1981; Best, 2008; Kitsuse and Cicourel, 1963; and, more recently, J. Best, 2001. Take, for example, the BMI (Body Mass Index) calculation, the central measure used to determine obesity. Many in the realm of public health and science recognize BMI as an imperfect, if not outright faulty, formula for determining obesity since it only measures height and weight and is unable to account for such important variables as nutritional intake, muscularity, or fat distribution. BMI thresholds have not only endured, but in 1998 they were lowered by the National Institute of Health, propelling many more adults into the category of overweight than previously registered. (The BMI designation of overweight was lowered from twenty-seven to twenty-five for women.) Scholars point out that BMI, as a measure of body mass, was never intended as a measure of obesity. It is an easy calculation, providing a quick snapshot. In the realm of public health, this makes quite a bit of sense as a crude means to track population change, but falls short for any other purpose. Some scholars have noted the low and arbitrary definitions of "overweight" and "obese," despite the fact that recent health research has suggested that those who are slightly overweight in late adulthood live longer than those at an optimal weight, even though mortality rates for

obese people remain significantly higher than for both these categories. Others have pointed out that we have a tendency to collapse thin and healthy because of our antifat bias. See Boero, 2012; Campos et al., 2006; and Saguy, 2012. The anthropological research on obesity suggests a much more ambiguous relationship between weight and mortality.

48 Biltekoff, 2013: 7.

49 C. Ogden, M. Lamb, and M. Carroll (2010), "Obesity and Socioeconomic Status in Children and Adolescents: United States, 2005–2008," NCHS Data Brief No. 51, http://www.cdc.gov.

50 United States Public Law 106–525 (2000), also called the "Minority Health and Health Disparities Research and Education Act," provides a legal definition for health disparities as follows: "A population is a health disparity population if there is a significant disparity in the overall rate of disease incidence, prevalence, morbidity, mortality or survival rates in the population as compared to the health status of the general population." http://www.ncbi.nlm.nih.gov (downloaded Jan. 4, 2014).

51 There is also a growing set of debates in physical anthropology around race as a social construct, epigenetics, the legacy of institutional racism, and health disparities. See for example Gravlee, 2009; Kuzawa and Sweet, 2009; Wells, 2012.

52 See Yale University's Rudd Center for Food Policy and Obesity's 2008 report "Access to Healthy Food in Low-Income Neighborhoods: Opportunities for Public Policy," http://www.ct.gov. See also Fitzpatrick and LaGory, 2000, as well as Wacquant, 2006.

53 Nestle, 2002.

54 See "Adolescent and School Health: Health Disparities," Centers for Disease Control, http://www.cdc.gov (downloaded Jan. 4, 2014). It is perhaps not surprising, then, that school would be identified as an important site for meaningful and productive intervention to close a health gap between poor children and middle- and upper-income children. Though schools as public institutions have long played an important role in the reproduction of social stratification, they have played an equally important role in attempting to mitigate social inequalities between families and communities by narrowing the gaps in opportunity and offsetting the stalled mobility of the disadvantaged and the marginalized.

55 For example Besen-Cassino (2014) notes that lower-income youth of color are virtually excluded from the high-demand service jobs that carry high status and brand recognition for youth, in part because these jobs are concentrated in upper-income suburban communities.

56 Harris, Schwartz, and Brownell, 2010: 10. In 2014 the Rudd Center moved to University of Connecticut.

57 See "Fast Food F.A.C.T.S.," *Grist*, 2010, http://grist.files.wordpress.com (downloaded Oct. 14, 2013).

58 Harris, Schwartz, and Brownell, 2013.

59 Harris, Schwartz, and Brownell, 2010.

60 Though importantly, in actuality they have never been fully separated spheres. See Cook, 2004; Zelizer, 2005.

61 See Texas Department of Agriculture, "School District Vending Contract Survey, 2003," March 24, 2005, www.squaremeals.org.

62 See "80 Percent of Public Schools Have Contracts with Coke or Pepsi," *Mother Jones*, Aug. 15, 2012, http://www.motherjones.com (downloaded Jan. 4, 2014).

63 Poppendeick, 2010.

64 Healthy eating practices are positively associated with a host of health outcomes. See Weaver-Hightower, 2011.

65 Most competitive foods' nutritional profile fails to meet federal dietary guidelines that determine whether a meal will be reimbursed by the government. The presence of revenue-generating foods, like Doritos, in schools, as Poppendieck (2010) has noted, ultimately drives down sales of reimbursable meals, which are healthier and more nutritionally balanced.

66 Under the 2010 Healthy and Hunger-Free Kids Act, competitive foods will be subject to some regulation.

67 Poppendieck, 2010: 4.

68 Historian Susan Levine (2008) notes that there has always been a disconnect between the public school lunchroom in practice and lunch on paper. The schism between the ideal of a school lunch program and its reality is perhaps nowhere more evident than in the fact that the National School Lunch Program, administered by the USDA, operated as government insurance policy for agriculture and did so for decades before the passage of the School Lunch Bill. The commodity distribution program, also run out of USDA, stabilized food prices by controlling supply of surplus farm produce. This was once a lifeline for farmers, but did little to ensure that foods high in nutritional value made it on the school menu. As Levine documents, the rise of food relief during the Depression era is a story about labor and livelihoods as much as it is about farm subsidies and commodity supports that led to what we now call industrial agriculture and the industrial diet. Many who advocate for food policy reform have argued that this creates a conflict of interest for USDA, since aims of healthy, nutritional food for all students irrespective of the ability to pay stands opposed to the interests of the agricultural industries' commodity program.

69 Today the NSLP must also compete against student groups: the entrepreneur club at one school studied sold cans of Coke for under a dollar. Another student club sold Krispy Kreme donuts to raise funds for its annual field trip. For food directors, the cafeteria must break even. Food directors face innumerable pressures to build revenues to offset operating costs, which explains the proliferation of à la carte offerings and snacks in the last twenty-five years.

70 2010: 2.

71 See "Special Report: How Washington Went Soft on Childhood Obesity," *Reuters*, April 27, 2012, http://www.reuters.com (downloaded Jan. 4, 2014).

72 See "DC Reject Soda Tax but Funds Better School Food," *Grist*, May 27, 2010, http://grist.org (downloaded Jan. 4, 2014).

73 Poppendieck, 2010: 100.

74 See "A Child's Day: 2009 Detailed Tables," U.S. Census Bureau, Aug. 11, 2011, http://www.census.gov. See also "Empty Seats: Few Families Eat Together," *Gallup*, Jan. 20, 2014, http://www.gallup.com.

75 Hochschild, 2003: 13.

76 See "Food Hardship in America," Food Research and Action Center, 2012, http://frac.org. Food Research and Action Center (FRAC) analyzes data that were collected by Gallup. The data were gathered as part of the Gallup-Healthways Well-Being Index project, which has been interviewing almost a thousand households daily since January 2008. FRAC has analyzed responses to the question, "Have there been times in the past twelve months when you did not have enough money to buy food that you or your family needed?" The report contains data throughout 2012 for every state, region, congressional district, and one hundred of the country's largest metropolitan areas (MSA).

77 See for example Patel's (2007) *Stuffed and Starved,* which documents the distinctly modern trend of hunger and obesity occurring simultaneously within the same poor communities across the globe and arising from a world food system that has concentrated power in the hands of a few Western corporations, has exacerbated global poverty, and has contributed to decline in the environment.

78 See, for example, Poppendieck's (1999) *Sweet Charity.*

79 1992.

80 2005.

81 This is based on the schools' demographic profiles in 2010.

82 In 2012, I observed eight additional public school cafeterias for another project. My observations from those schools informed my thinking, but are not used as data for this project.

83 In a context of food abundance, the way we use foods provides us with clues about the cultural currency of the body as instrumental object, love object, moral object, and aesthetic object.

CHAPTER 1. THE FAMILY MEAL

1 1997.

2 Douglas, 1972.

3 Lupton, 1994.

4 Bell and Valentine, 1997: Johnston and Cairns, 2015; DeVault, 1991; James, Curtis, and Ellis, 2009; Kaplan, 2000.

5 See James, Curtis, and Ellis, 2009.

6 1991.

7 2003: 2. Much has been made of, for example, the sandwich generation, a generation of women who must provide care for their children while also caring for aging parents, who are living longer but are often without the range of resources

to do so. Hochschild (1997) suggests in her book *The Time Bind* that the rise of blended families and the increased demands of familial care at a historical period when time is divided increasingly between work and home has contributed to a sense of family as work.

8 Hochschild, 1997: 2003.

9 Nestle, 2002; Patel, 2007; Pollen, 2007; Winson, 2013.

10 Bianchi, Robinson, and Milkie (2007), drawing on time-use diaries, have argued that increases in workable hours is uneven. While some households have experienced a significant ratcheting up of hours, other workers have been subject to declining hours. The result is "too much work at some stages of life and too little work at others" (39).

11 Bianchi, Robinson, and Milkie, 2007.

12 Berk, 2005: 20. Parents' income and education correlate with children's participation rates in extracurricular/organized activities, with higher levels of participation among higher-income families with college or advanced degrees, according to the "A Child's Day," U.S. Census (http://www.census.gov). This has also been demonstrated in ethnographic accounts, such as Annette Lareau's *Unequal Childhoods* (2003). Lareau details time-use differences among children by class and examines the class logics that explain it.

13 Stacey, 1997.

14 Andrew Cherlin (2009) has identified transformations in family forms as triggered by a deinstitutionalization of marriage, evidenced by a weakening of social norms that define and guide behavior in family and marriage. These norm changes have been linked to (1) changing division of labor and roles in marriage, (2) increase in childrearing outside marriage, (3) rising rates of cohabitation, and (4) the emergence of same-sex marriage and blended family forms. Madonna Harrington Meyer (2007) has shown the lasting economic impact of declining marriage rates for aging women, for example.

15 Pugh, 2015. This is also a theme explored by Eva Illouz (2007).

16 See also Giddens, 1991.

17 Poppendieck, 2010: 100.

18 Child Trends also reports that adolescents cite interest in autonomy, scheduling conflicts, and family discord as reasons for the decline in shared meals times, while parents cite time demands and conflicting schedules as being responsible. See Child Trends, "Family Meal: Indicators on Children and Youth," May 2013, www.childtrend.org (downloaded July 26, 2016).

19 Source: U.S. Census Bureau, "Survey of Income and Program Participation," 2008 Panel, Wave 4, August 2010, https://www.census.gov. The U.S. Census reports that parents with lower monthly incomes are more likely to report eating dinner with their 12–17-year-old child daily than parents with higher monthly incomes. Those who own homes are less likely to report eating with their 12–17-year-old child daily than those who rent. Those who receive government food assistance are more likely to report eating dinner with their

12–17-year-old child daily than parents who don't receive food assistance. See "A Child's Day: 2009 Detailed Tables," U.S. Census Bureau, Aug. 11, 2011, https://www.census.gov. For lower-income families during much of the first half of the twentieth century, "[P]roper family meals were unheard of, and food was simply left on a bare table for family members to grab when they could" (Shapiro, 1986: 130).

20 See U.S. Census Bureau, "A Child's Day: 2009 Detailed Tables," Aug. 11, 2011, https://www.census.gov.

21 Changes in family meals are generally recognized as important because of the value we culturally attach to the family; shared family meals are often regarded as a measure of family well-being.

22 Historians remind us that work patterns have long impinged upon family patterns of food consumption. Cinotto writes,

> Much of the ceremonialism that the Victorian middle class attached to food consumption concentrated on dinner, which, to accommodate urban work and school schedules, gradually moved from midday to evening. In the late nineteenth century, the increasingly suburban middle-class families finally ate dinner at seven o'clock, when commuting men had returned home. The ritual significance of dinner derived from its status as the only time of the day when all the family gathered in the presence of the father: the less time the family spent together, the more important that little time became. (Cinotto, 2006: 20–21)

23 Marjorie DeVault (1991) has argued that family scholars have paid insufficient attention to the specific activities that constitute family life and in so doing, inadvertently naturalize and normalize particular family forms, roles, and arrangements. DeVault's (1991) research documenting the invisible work of feeding the family, largely undertaken by women, draws attention to the particular activities and routines that constitute family life. DeVault's research zeroes in on the symbolic terrain of food and women's activities in creating this terrain; her emphasis on the essentially processual and contingent nature of these family activities and rituals is a useful framework for thinking about family life as a routine, interactional, and collaborative achievement. Her research demonstrates the importance of this work to constructing and maintaining family connections. DeVault shows how the physical tasks of food preparation combine with the work of connection and sociability to produce group life in households.

24 The interviews with youth aged fifteen to eighteen provide support that the nostalgia around family and food that will be discussed in the pages that follow is not simply a consequence of life stage and circumstance for this group of writers who now are in college, since similar themes emerged around food and family across age groups. It is also important to note that while college students are typically thought to live away from home and parents during college and thus may feel particularly nostalgic for family and home food, a large percentage of students at the state university where this sample was drawn continued to live at home. Taken

together, these two points suggest that the sentimentalism identified in young people's accounts of family and food is not simply a consequence of their physical distance from home as they begin to transition to adulthood.

25 This chapter draws heavily on the conceptual framing of family life as shaped by processes of marketization as articulated by Arlie Hochschild (2003), who identifies as significant to the arrangement of daily family life a growing care gap, whereby the delivery of care by intimate others in group settings has been transformed by external constraints arising from the ever-increasing time demands of work under a system of advanced capitalism, a system characterized by a high level of worker insecurity, while also thought responsible for ushering a market logic (e.g., the speeding up of home life and focus on the efficient delivery of care) into the familial sphere.

26 Cinotto, 2006: 24.

27 Narrative #172. Each narrative is numbered and footnoted in order for the reader to see how consistent the themes were across the 260 plus written narratives. Individuals who were interviewed were given a fictional name. The written narratives were numbered.

28 Narrative #130.

29 Narrative #71.

30 Narrative #15.

31 Narrative #18.

32 Narrative #77.

33 Narrative #16.

34 Narrative #178.

35 Narrative #87.

36 Narrative #9.

37 Narrative #267.

38 Narrative #13.

39 Narrative #174.

40 Narrative #65.

41 Narrative #31.

42 Narrative #94.

43 Narrative #6.

44 Narrative #261.

45 Hochschild, 1997.

46 Narrative #91.

47 Narrative #62.

48 Narrative #34.

49 Narratives #67, #94.

50 Narrative #27.

51 Narrative #213.

52 Narrative #6.

53 Narrative #175.

54 It is interesting that the absence of the father indicates a fractured family, suggesting that traditional ideas about father as head of household may still be in play. However, I also found that young writers noted the absence of older siblings and mothers as well.

55 Narrative #128.

56 Narrative #158.

57 Narrative #31.

58 Narrative #79.

59 Narrative #143.

60 Narrative #154.

61 Narrative #69.

62 See Brembeck, 2009, for a discussion of immigrant youth and family food.

63 Narrative #148.

64 Narrative #66. Emphasis in the original.

65 Narrative #121.

66 Narrative #140.

67 Narrative #158.

68 Narrative #193.

69 Narrative #48.

70 Narrative #41.

71 Narrative #117.

72 Narrative #59.

73 Narrative #85.

74 Narrative #159.

75 Narrative #130.

76 Eid, the feast of breaking fast, marks the end of Ramadan, and Diwali, a Hindu festival of lights, is celebrated in the fall.

77 Hochschild, 2003: 16.

78 Narrative #35.

79 Narrative #70.

80 Narrative # 32.

81 Narrative #42.

82 Narrative #25.

83 Narrative #49.

84 Narrative #70.

85 Narrative #111.

86 Narrative #48.

87 Narrative #29.

88 2004: 44.

89 Narrative #62.

90 Narrative #91.

91 Sociologist Amitai Etzioni (2004) opines, "In a society that has made economic advancement a key value while downgrading others, people dedicate more and

more of their time to work and commerce, and less to family, community, and holidays" (3). Yet, what is clear from these youth is that *greater* significance is attached to family holidays, *not less*, precisely because of the time given over to work and pursuits outside the family sphere.

92 2003: 39.

93 Narrative #168.

94 Narrative #97.

95 Narrative #56.

96 For those writers whose mothers cooked, they were able to align the routine activities of their mothers with an order of ceremony and sentimentalism. In the language of Goffman, obligation and expectation are in perfect balance and so too is the prevailing moral order. As community supports erode under the weight of economic demands, the mother is increasingly idealized as a figure of love and support. Hochschild (2003) writes, "The hypersymbolization of the mother is itself partly a response to the destabilization of the cultural as well as economic ground on which the family rests" (39).

97 See Food Research and Action Center, "National School Lunch Program," http://frac.org (downloaded July 25, 2016).

98 Narrative #125.

99 Narrative #176.

100 Marj DeVault's (1991) work on feeding the family demonstrates that meal preparation shapes a whole complex of relations—wife-husband, mother-child—solidifying gender and feminine deference in husband and wife relations into distinct forms.

101 Narrative #155. While mothers took center stage, fathers were either absent from the food memories, background actors, or acknowledged but cast in supporting roles, with the exception of father's kitchen escapades as a kind of comic relief. Thomas Adler explains that when men cook in the home, it is deciphered through a different lexicon of meaning. "Any regular pattern of male cookery probably contains some elements of a symbolic inversion. Dad's cooking exists in evident contradistinction to Mom's on every level: his is festal, hers ferial; his is socially and gastronomically experimental, hers mundane; his is dish-specific and temporally marked, hers diversified and quotidian; his is play, hers is work" (Adler, 1981: 51). In the data I collected, father's cooking was characterized as "a rare treat" (#45) and tended to focus on a single food item, e.g., "My dad's chocolate milk shake" (#127).

102 Narrative #125.

103 Narrative #18.

104 Narrative #56.

105 Narrative #141.

106 Narrative #34.

107 Narrative #131.

108 Narrative #116. But in this writer's case, as he and his sister grew older, more time was spent away from family, and dinners together became less frequent. Since the

majority of his meals are now taken out, the shared Sunday meal, as a locus of family unity, has shifted back to the home, is once again traditional Indian fare, and is prepared by his mother and sister.

109 Narrative #123.

110 Miller, 2001: 109.

111 Narrative #27.

112 Narrative #218.

113 Narrative #149.

114 Cook, 2009: 115.

115 Commercial foods, in these accounts, then, occupied a rather ambiguous place, on the one hand cast in sharp contrast to the sentimental world of family life embodied in home-cooked food, and on the other hand, a part of meaningful family memories. Sociologist Viviana Zelizer (2005) argues,

> In the commercialized United States of the early twenty-first century, household members still remain the principal providers of care to other household members. No doubt that household concentration of caring services reinforces the supposition of a sharp division between the diffuse, sentimental, and non-commercial world of the family and the specialized, impersonal and commercialized world of goods and services outside the family. (172)

116 See Pew Social Trends, "The Decline of Marriage and Rise of New Families," Nov. 11, 2010, http://www.pewsocialtrends.org.

117 Rationalization and consumerism have reorganized cultural fields once thought to be impenetrable by commercial influence, most notably for this analysis, the family. See Ritzer, 2005; Hochschild, 1997, 2003.

118 2006: 19.

119 2006: 17. Cinotto also noted that "as the functions of the family became mostly psychological and ideological, family rituals became more important" (20).

120 1929: 153–54.

121 1992: 2.

122 2003: 2.

123 2003: 35.

124 Hochschild, 2003: 35.

125 As Maurice Halbwachs (1992), who developed the concept of collective memory, famously argued, memory is a selective social phenomenon, dependent on the collective context of its construction and articulation. More recently Alison Landsberg (2004) has written on what she has called "prosthetic memory," created by new technologies of memory (such as film) such that memory emerges as a mass-produced commodity. Prosthetic memories are memories "originating outside a person's lived experience and yet are taken on and worn by that person through mass-mediated cultural technology of memory. . . . [T]hey [memories] derive from a person's mass-mediated experience" (19). "Commodification," Landsberg adds, "enables memory and images of the past to circulate on a grand scale," making possible "new modalities of subjectivity and new structure of feelings" (18).

126 1992.

127 Bianchi, Robinson, and Milkie, 2007.

128 2003: 165.

129 2003: 23.

CHAPTER 2. THE CAFETERIA AS GREAT EQUALIZER

1 Both are district food directors, but I focus in this book specifically on the work they did for the high schools where I observed.

2 2008: 12.

3 Levine, 2008.

4 Levine (2008) notes that in the original signing of the School Lunch Bill there were no provisions made to ensure compliance, making it difficult for the federal government to ensure states would match funds, a requirement of the bill, or guarantee that children who most stood to benefit from free lunches were able to participate in the program. (Cumbersome paperwork to apply for and determine eligibility for free or reduced lunch, for example, kept thousands of eligible children from participating in the program in the 1980s and 1990s.) This was to continue over several decades as parents came to provide increasing support for lunch programs. Levine notes that most states ignored the free-lunch mandate well through the 1960s so that most children did not receive a free lunch.

5 Levine, 2008: 110.

6 Levine, 2008: 145.

7 Poppendieck, 2010: 130. The amount of the subsidy depends on income qualification. All children who purchase lunch through the National School Lunch Program are subsidized by the federal government at twenty-six cents. For families whose income falls below 135 percent of the poverty line, lunch is free. This means that the federal government will provide a $2.72 reimbursement to the school for the cost of lunch as long it meets the federal nutritional guidelines. For families above the 135 percent but below 185 percent above the poverty line, lunch is reduced. Today, those who qualify for free or reduced lunch receive the same food through the National School Lunch Program as those who don't qualify but are usually excluded from the purchase of competitive foods (also called à la carte food items).

8 Nestle, 2002.

9 Gosliner et al., 2011.

10 2010.

11 See Center for Science in the Public Interest, http://www.cspinet.org (downloaded July 27, 2016).

12 See Campaign for a Commercial-Free Childhood, http://commercialfreechildhood.org (downloaded July 27, 2016).

13 See Corporate Accountability International, http://www.stopcorporateabuse.org (downloaded July 27, 2016).

14 Many school administrators and PTAs, especially those in poor districts, have historically welcomed, often with open arms, the food industry and its attendant marketing because they offer improved revenue and resources for the school. To say no is to turn a collective back on "free money."

15 To qualify for reduced lunch under the federal program in 2012, a family of four cannot have total earnings that exceed $39,000. To qualify for free lunch a family of four cannot have total earning exceeding $27,000.

16 Food Research Action Center recently reported, on the basis of a 2012 U.S. Gallup's Healthways and Well-being Index, that one in six Americans reports being food insecure—which is defined as having struggled to feed their families during the previous twelve months. See Food Research Action Center, "Food Hardship in America 2012," Feb. 2013, http://frac.org.

17 I am not sure why they do not accept them.

18 These percentages are based on the period of observation in 2010.

19 If off-campus privileges are granted, it will probably mean that those kids who can pay for lunch off campus will, and those left behind will be kids on free or reduced lunch. It is the case that even kids who qualify for free or reduced lunch might forego opportunity for an in-school lunch, a lunch that meets the dietary guidelines, in favor of a bag of chips bought off campus. Many advocates and policy workers focused on free and reduced lunch have noted that some students will opt out of NSLP to avoid risk of the stigma of "free lunch." This causes obvious problems. In the case of Thurgood, I observed some degree of openness about a student's status as free- or reduced-lunch eligible. Though it was not entirely commonplace, I did observe some kids say openly, "I'm free." At Washington, where the percentage of free- or reduced-lunch eligible is much, much smaller, I expect the stigma to be magnified. I never observed a single student openly discuss his or her lunch status.

20 Signaling broader trends in the business of school food sales and production, the cafeteria's design is consistent with the branding recommendations food directors receive at national food conferences (Poppendieck, 2010).

21 The U.S. Department of Labor reports that nearly 40 percent of food dollars for American households are spent on food eaten away from home and that nearly 60 percent of Americans will eat a meal or snack away from home on any given day. Half of Americans' daily calories are derived from food eaten outside the home. See Agricultural Research Service, U.S. Department of Agriculture, "Food Away from Home," Oct. 2014, http://www.ars.usda.gov. See also Poti and Popkin, 2011, on the role eating location plays in energy intake.

22 There is some research that lends empirical support to the claim that commercial food companies purposely open food outlets near schools to tap youth markets. See Austin et al., 2005.

23 The school's kitchen is the central kitchen for the whole district.

24 Massengill, 2013: 5.

25 See Rios, 2012, and Warikoo, 2013.

26 This example speaks to how fraught "choice" as a concept can be since it can be utilized for such drastically different ends.

27 See, for example, Jonathan Kozol's *Savage Inequalities* (1991), *The Shame of the Nation: The Restoration of Apartheid Schooling in America* (2005), and *Fire in the Ashes: Twenty-Five Years among the Poorest Children in America* (2012). In 2011, I attended a chef cook-off in an urban public charter high school in celebration of the national Farm to School week in one of the poorest neighborhoods in the city. A new building, it was clean, bright, and orderly. Of course, just beyond its locked doors was a sidewalk peppered with empty whiskey bottles and beer cans, crumpled bags of chips, and cigarette butts. As one of the chefs came into the building and then the gym, he looked around, and with a sardonic tone of surprise, remarked, "This is much nicer than the suburban high school I attended."

28 Family poverty and parental absence were often offered as explanation for a host of problems students faced.

29 In Penelope Eckert's classic *Jocks and Burnouts*, the working-class kids who smoked cigarettes and occupied space on the perimeter of school rejected cafeteria food wholesale, claiming it had made friends sick. Eckert persuasively argues that the Burnouts' rejection of cafeteria food was in fact a rejection of the school's disingenuous attempt to play a parental role.

30 This contrasts with some of the elementary school cafeterias I observed for a project of farm-to-school programming, where significant plate waste was generated. While at Washington, by my estimate, maybe one-third of the kids brought lunch from home on any given day; at Thurgood, I saw only a handful of kids with lunch from home at each lunch each day. (A whole host of reasons determine why kids eat lunch in the cafeteria, a point to be addressed in the next chapter.)

31 Brenda was actually particularly critical of the chefs' movement to transform school lunch, in part I suspect because of the sense of scrutiny she had felt and the sense of belittling of her profession and occupational status. Referring to the chefs' movement, she had this to offer:

> Didn't help us at all. It opened a conversation which I guess can be a positive way but my own personal philosophy is when you speak from a bully pulpit you're speaking from a position of power. . . . When you say school lunch is terrible you've never been to my program, you don't know my program. You don't know every district in this country is different . . . unique needs, different budgets . . . [A]s a whole, as a group of professional people, we have a passion for this. I've been in this work for over twenty years. I wouldn't be here if I didn't care and care deeply and so it really offends me when people are ill informed and don't know even a little bit but worse still don't bother to ask and just say, you know, you should do all fresh cooking. You should all do this, you should do that and it can be done in certain places but you still have to work incrementally to make change and unfortunately people don't always want to see that. . . . It's hard work and it's worthwhile work. I'm

not in it to gain celebrity . . . [W]hen you look at websites and you see that people, out of their districts X number of days out of the month, I don't get paid to be out of my district. I get paid to serve the children in my district and so that's just my little bias you know and that's probably incorrect politically but I'm at the age where I can say what I think.

This tension reflects two professional groups, chefs and nutritionists, in some sense belonging to separate camps, struggling over the symbolic boundaries of professional worth and value of work. That the head cook at one school I visited for this project carries the title Chef Sara is instructive and no doubt an effort to symbolically elevate the work and occupation, since neither is given its ceremonial due.

32 This is precisely what happened in a neighboring school district. High-sugar flavored milks were removed and replaced with low-sugar flavored milk. This lasted about six months before the school district was able to arrive at a better compromise and found a flavored milk with less sugar and few added antibiotics, but more sugar than the first.

33 Brenda also explained, "I don't look at one food as one particular nutrient. I look at the profile of the food, also the research." Statements such as the following were common in the interview: "The research shows you have to put it out ten or twelve times anyway but here because we do some stuff over and over that happens faster, um, I think when I've talked to kids I think they would say that."

34 Goffman's seminal work on the stigma is instructive. To be sure, poverty is a discreditable stigma, not immediately obvious in social encounters.

35 Brenda recognized the limits of her powers: "[W]hat we don't do well is integrate nutrition education throughout the curriculum. . . . What we don't do well is to enable children to learn about the love of food and the love of socializing across a meal."

36 Brenda explains,

There's an economy of scale. There's a few all-reduced-eligible children. By law we could charge them forty cents for lunch, up to forty cents and up to thirty cents for breakfast. About thirteen or fourteen years ago the school board decided that upon the recommendation of the food service director at the time that we would give those children free meals so what that means is that we have to make up that forty cents. . . . So we get the reduced rate to us.

As the demographic of school has shifted toward a greater number of high-need students, this has become an increasingly costly proposition.

37 Interestingly, Brenda did remark that the teachers and staff, many black themselves, expressed greater appreciation for the southern soul food offering than the kids.

38 Mead also promoted foods with "low emotional value" (Levine, 2008: 68), concerned that foods tied to ethnic or national origins might exacerbate divisions or alienate one group from another.

39 In the interview Brenda addressed this issue:

I feel like I educate them. . . . First thing they say is we want more healthy food so when they say healthy food, I say well, we need to be on the same wavelength. I need to understand what you think is healthy because I know what I serve is healthy . . . so I'll pull out the menu, and I said well did you see we had twenty-five and thirty different fresh fruits or vegetables?

40 See, for example, ypulse, an organization focused on youth marketing that has a significant online presence. Available at http://www.ypulse.com (downloaded July 27, 2016).

41 This, of course has policy implications. Policy and practice that thrive in one setting, only to find a wall of difficulty in another, present a genuine quagmire for policy makers working to implement food and educational change across school settings.

42 Marketplace relations and the consumer experiences for youth of color are fraught. Too often they are treated with little respect as customers, especially when venturing into retail settings where they are thought to be interlopers. See, for instance, Zukin, 2003: "Artemio Goes to Tiffany's."

43 Her efforts did not pass unnoticed. The school was awarded first place for best kids' menu by a trade magazine for restaurant and hospitality industries.

44 See, for example, FONA International, "Not a Millennial but I'm Still Worth Watching: Who Am I? Generation Z," 2016 Trend Insight Report, www.fona.com.

45 Other school districts serve ethnic foods as part of multicultural educational enrichment.

46 That access to healthy food must also be accompanied by nutritional education was a point both food directors acknowledged. Both recognized the importance of nutritional education, suggesting that parents and children stand to benefit from greater food literacy. "I try to really work with parents. On our website we do nutrition education articles. We do a little blurb on our menus for elementary that talk about various nutrition topics." But both also recognize their failure in that regard. Brenda recognized the limits of her powers: "[W]hat we don't do well is integrate nutrition education throughout the curriculum. . . . What we don't do well is to enable children to learn about the love of food and the love of socializing across a meal." Thurgood did have a successful culinary arts program run by a professionally trained chef who was very well liked by the students. Its focus as an elective, however, was on professional training for students who are considering moving into food service and was less on nutritional education.

CHAPTER 3. THE CAFETERIA AS YOUTH SPACE

1 Theft by consolidation was also a point Brenda raised in the interview, though she attributed theft by consolidation to the issue of food insecurity and hunger.

2 Unlike at Washington, I recorded very few instances of kids with commercial foods. I saw once a boy with a McDonald's bag, on another day a girl with a Chipotle bag, but little else. One day, a group of girls shared a store-bought birthday cake.

3 Apart from the bathrooms, that is. The historian William Graebner (1990) points out that the bathroom has long been one of the few unsupervised and thus more autonomous spaces in school, which helps to explain why limits are often placed on how many are permitted in the bathroom at one time and for how long.

4 See Graebner, 1990.

5 Years ago when I was observing in high schools for an ethnography on high school proms, at one of the urban public high schools, long benches were placed at the entrance to the cafeteria to barricade the exit (an obvious fire code violation).

6 Eckert (1989) also observed this dilemma in her observation at schools.

7 At Washington High School, the small number of Spanish-speaking immigrant youth from Central and South America always sat together at a table in the farthest corner of the room, while at Thurgood, where white students were in the minority, many sat together each day at two large tables in the middle of the room, quietly talking.

8 1997: 30.

9 2010.

10 There is some disconnect between Thurgood and the community where it resides. There were identified tensions between the community where Thurgood is located (an older and very expensive part of the city) and the school itself, which tends to draw students from other areas of the city represented by low-income families, many immigrants, and African Americans. The city population is 23 percent black and 56 percent white, non-Hispanic, 25 percent foreign born. Eight percent of households fall below the poverty line. Children living below the poverty threshold are 17 percent for the city. Wealthy students largely attend private schools. There are several reputable private schools in the city. Only 14 percent of households have children. The school district has a substantial budget with per-pupil spending considerably higher than in neighboring districts.

11 The school has grappled with charges of racial sorting, yet a narrative of overcoming racial segregation is central to the way the school understands itself. A 1971 desegregation injunction led to the school's integration. In the early 1970s, the school led the state in integrating its student population. Demographic change in both city and school since the 1970s led to a dramatic increase in the percentage of students living in low-income housing, many food insecure. A growing number of students are from immigrant families, and the number of squarely middle-class families living within the school district has declined, as property values around the school have skyrocketed. In this way the school might be recognized as trending toward what journalist Jonathon Kozol has recently termed schooling "resegregation." The school's history of desegregation and current racial diversity was a source of school pride, but in fact the school is highly segregated, with a racial split visible in sports, the classroom, and the cafeteria. See also Orfield, Eaton, and the Harvard Project on School Desegregation, 1998, as well as Troutt, 2014.

12 In the mid-2000s, the school received some negative press after a student-generated survey revealing race-based academic tracking by teachers and guidance counselors was presented to the press. The dropout rate hovers between 10 and 13 percent, and the vast majority of dropouts are minority. Race is ever present at this school. Race is sometimes named explicitly but more often than not is talked about in a coded language—in terms of food ("our kind of food") or academics (white kids overrepresented in AP tracks). It was often conflated with class-free subsidized lunch, community disorganization, and "fragmented homes." These are flag terms used to discuss persistent poverty. I can also recall talking with a substitute teacher during one lunch period who told me he normally taught as a substitute in a higher-income school thirty miles from Thurgood; the kids were "really affluent"; "some of them are amazing," he told me with traces of excitement in his voice. But "in a place like this . . . just trying to prevent them from killing each other" is a challenge, he said.

13 Citation is withheld to protect the confidentiality of the school.

14 However, another study found that in the 2006–2007 year, only 17 percent of all students participated in AP classes, a lower percentage than in neighboring schools. This study also found that race patterns enrollment in AP classes, with 50 percent white and only 9 percent black, 14 percent Asian, and 6 percent Latino similarly enrolled. The same study found that while 63 percent of whites graduated with an advanced diploma, a requirement for entrance to many colleges, only 10 percent black and 15 percent Latino students did. Citation is withheld to protect the confidentiality of the school.

15 They hired a new principal and nearly seventy new staff, while firing a large number of long-term teachers. In fact, 50 percent of the staff had been hired in the last three years. While a number of the administrators with whom I spoke remarked that they were under a lot of pressure because of this label, there was also a tangible sense of change. I do not have space here to analyze the labor politics of teachers and mass terminations in large public school, but this is a meaningful issue that deserves attention elsewhere.

16 In the preceding several years, there had been a steady rotation of leadership, as the district had worked to address the problem in academic achievement. As Jacob, a student I interviewed who had graduated from Thurgood two years earlier, remarked, "They've been going through superintendents and principals like the Redskins do coaches." But Vice Principal Edwards told me that the new principal "gets things done." The new rules were not met with a warm welcome by all students, of course. In one interview, the changes were characterized as "cracking down," with a shift from a "laissez-faire approach to the students" to "security cameras everywhere," "closed campus now."

17 After 2010, the school hired a dean of students for each grade.

18 This is particularly meaningful in light of the youth social movement mobilized against what is often called "the school-to-prison pipeline" and the specific target-

ing and criminalization of boys of color through punitive school policies. See Ferguson, 2001, for an excellent discussion of these dynamics.

19 See, for example, Tilton's (2010) excellent discussion of the racially charged dimension of public schooling in Oakland, California, and white, middle-class retreat from public institutions.

20 Cool and school are often cast at odds. Consider, for instance, the popular singer Pink's "Raise Your Glass" lyrics: "If you're too school for cool."

21 In fact, the school had identified, as an important strategic intervention in the achievement gap, stronger relationship development between faculty and staff and the students.

22 Much of the one-to-one work focused on black kids. I saw far fewer exchanges with Latinos, many of whom are ESL.

23 I observed many examples of working to connect with students meaningfully. One morning I arrived at the cafeteria before lunch had begun. They were in their last hour of a workshop they were running on post–high school. A portion was dedicated to applying to college and another portion to preparing a resume for post–high school employment. I was struck by the tone of all the speakers, a mix of teachers and student deans, as they addressed the students. There was widespread acknowledgment that students might not already possess this knowledge from home and parents—that they were imparting this knowledge because they wanted to help students succeed and thought a number of the student should go on to college. Students were repeatedly thanked for being courteous and attentively listening. Specific advice was given to students about how to write a compelling personal statement when applying to college. The speaker provided as an example a successful essay by a former student who wrote about how he worked at a bakery three hours every morning before coming to school in order to help support his family.

24 1967.

25 This stands in contrast to Washington, where adults were all but absent in the cafeteria and certainly did not engage the same interactional work undertaken here. I borrow this term from Allison Pugh (2009), who discusses dignity work on children's peer interactions, where consumer goods figure centrally.

26 See, for example, Rios, 2012; Tilton, 2010; Wacquant, 2010.

27 See Victor Turner's seminal work on liminality (1969).

28 Jodi Miller (2008) uses the term "contested play claims" to describe the competing gendered interpretations of boys' and girls' actions where play and more troubling behavior are debated.

29 Miller (2008) makes the point that girls face a higher risk of violence in disadvantaged neighborhoods because of high levels of social isolation of and within these neighborhoods and because of barriers to developing collective community efficacy.

30 Miller, 2008: 70–73. Jones (2010), in Between Good and Ghetto, also details the gendered violence girls encounter in community schools marked by urban disadvantage

31 See Lopez, *Hopeful Girls, Troubled Boys*, for a discussion of discipline and the racial logic of urban schooling. Clay, 2012; Rios, 2012

32 A few weeks into my observing at Washington, I noticed a small group of students as they moved through the lunch line because these always lingered and they always spoke Spanish to the ladies who worked the lunch line, exchanging warm greetings and engaging in small talk with them. They were ESL students, I learned from Joe.

33 For the most part, racial groupings at Washington were much less observable; most of the tables were racially mixed, with the exception of a group of all-white juniors, who typically claimed several tables at the center of the room, and a much smaller group of ESL students. Every day they claimed a spot at the farthest table in the corner of the long room, which also happened to be the table closest to the doorway to the back kitchen and which lunch ladies and custodial staff, most of whom were also Spanish speaking, used often. Watching these kids linger in the lunch line, talking in Spanish, exchanging warm greetings, and engaging in small talk with the lunch ladies, I often wondered if the lunch ladies were one of the more important institutional connections for these students. Joe told me that school was very hard for these kids. They were in the same room all day, it is hard to learn to speak English, and their opportunities for contact with other teachers and students were limited.

34 Usually an administrator would be camped out nearby since the assumption held by the administrative staff was that active gang recruitment occurred during lunch.

35 It is worth noting that by 2015, Hispanic student represented the largest racial-ethnic group at the school, at 37 percent.

36 Her book focuses primarily on middle-school-aged kids and less on high-school-aged ones.

37 Jacob noted the deep racial division at the school, manifest in classrooms, sports, the geography of the lunchroom, and friendship groups. "If there were like black people around that I'd met and was friends with then I would talk to them but if I was in the cafeteria I wasn't just about to go sit down next to some group that I'd never met and strike them up in conversation."

38 Zerubavel, 1984: 14.

39 On one occasion I watched a vice principal lightly reprimand a girl for climbing over the table and bench (this was the same girl whom I had watched yell at another vice principal in an earlier lunch). She responded, "Okay," eking out a forced apology. She left and returned with a juice, and I watched as she climbed over the bench, past a girl, and took her seat. For students this seemed an effort to avoid having to ask someone to move, finding it easier to go around.

40 See, for example, Tilton's (2010) discussion of these dynamics in gentrifying Oakland.

41 Jacob elaborated this point more fully:

I can definitely understand why they would do that, if I was in their position I would probably wind up doing the same thing too, just because I can go home and I have parents who care, who will make me do homework, who will help me with whatever studying I have, the other kids don't so I don't really blame the school for that. I definitely felt like that was the case but you know what are you going to do?

We certainly can trouble some of Jacob's remarks. The idea that helping or not helping with homework is an expression of parental care ignores the complex set of factors that shape parents' relationship to their children's school and its curriculum (language barriers, work demands, insufficient academic preparation to assist) or the variable ways parents express care that are not academic in focus.

42 I think we might also draw from Lareau's insights about the emerging sense of entitlement among the professional middle class as they interact within various institutional settings. An emerging sense of ambivalence seems to emerge alongside entitlement.

43 See Murray Milner's (2004) *Freaks, Geeks, and Cool Kids.*

44 Reay et al., 2008.

45 This meaning held very little currency at Washington, in large part because less than 8 percent of the kids were on free or subsidized lunch. A larger number of students brought lunch from home at Washington. On any given day, somewhere between one-third and one-half of the kids could be seen with the brown paper bags that signal outside lunch. Washington had a microwave to accommodate outside lunches, enabling students to reheat the meals brought, often the previous night's diner.

46 Robert and Weaver Hightower, 2011: 4.

47 For kids in advanced academic tracks, who run the risk of being labeled goody-two-shoes, social spaces such as the cafeteria can be problematic and thus, it is easier to pass below the radar or hover above it.

48 There was a widespread perception of parental absenteeism and families barely getting by. I heard again and again from administrators, "These kids don't want to go home." Teenagers will often delay time spent in school because school represents as much a social as an academic space. Yet, I do think it likely that for some students school may be a better place, clean and orderly in comparison to community and home. What I came to realize is the extent to which the administration ultimately saw poverty and its attendant problems as *the* explanatory variable for all behaviors and all actions.

CHAPTER 4. EAT WHAT'S GOOD FOR YOU

1 Vera Bradley, enormously popular among middle and high school girls, are quilted fabric bags, usually in floral patterns, and are mostly associated with a contemporary preppy youth cultural style. A lunch tote costs between twenty-five and forty dollars. Larger bags, such as the printed duffle bags, popular for car-

rying sports and dance equipment, usually cost between sixty and one hundred dollars.

2 Poppendieck (2010) reports that about 35 percent of high schools are either fully open campuses, allowing all students to come and go, or are partially open, whereby some students are free to leave campus.

3 I sometimes observed kids work to project a self as one who has fun, laughing loudly and dramatically, for what seemed the benefit of others beyond a specific table, but mostly students confined their interaction to those at their table.

4 These percentages are based on the period of observation in 2010.

5 It took me months to get an appointment with the principal and food director at Washington, but I eventually gained access and was more or less free to come and go for the two-month period before the school year ended.

6 Recognizing that in truth, these food types overlap considerably. Home-based food is often market-based food, as is school food.

7 Biltekoff, 2013: 99.

8 I often wondered if Dan had been hired precisely because he did not have a long history as a school food director.

9 Though how some students built their salads might raise an eyebrow.

10 Changes to the way cheese steak sandwiches were prepared provided one example. Previously the food service workers toasted the bun with the meat and cheese already on it. This turned the meat green. Though doing so was less efficient, Dan required that the meat and cheese be placed on the bun after it was toasted. The result was a more appealing cheese steak sandwich that students ate and I did too.

11 Food service workers in school are some of the lowest-paid workers in the United States, with wages that are miserably poor. Both Brenda and Dan were very respectful toward the food service workers. Neither was in a position to improve their wages, which meant the children of these food service workers probably qualified for the same free and reduced lunch they served. But what Dan did do was to encourage the workers to exercise some control over their work. They had some autonomy and were encouraged to innovate, and they did so. In one instance, Dan told me that a few of the food service workers had bought a book to teach themselves how to make fruit sculptures to entice the kids to marvel at and eat the fruit. "They took the initiative to do it," Dan explained with a tone of noted pride.

12 See Johnston and Baumann, 2015. Dan was in the process of phasing out Pop-Tarts, a favorite among students but high in calories. He referred to them as "emergency food."

13 On one occasion Dan and I chatted about marketing, and he remarked about how misleading it can be. He gave the example of a vendor who said he could sell soup for six cents per serving, but then Dan found out that the serving size was two ounces. "That's a gulp, not a serving."

14 Dan sought to create various partnerships to minimize budget shortfalls. He described

> slowly working my way into the whole community where we will provide meals for summer camp programs, provide it to the city, uh, eventually I would like to have people come and, I've done meals so that they have like father and son dinners and stuff like that. . . . I'm sure but you have people look at school food differently.

Imagining for a moment the unknown down the road, he said,

> I would like to do cartoons that promote healthy eating uh and commercials at the high school level. . . . [M]y ideal scenario, is to make this more like a food social environment. When people think the cafeteria is not just that place down the hall, when they think of food they think of us first, and we're getting there.

15 Pop-Tarts, he told me, would be phased out. Their current supply, a leftover from the year, would not be replenished.

16 While Brenda talked about PTA and the uptick in e-mail from parents in the preceding year as media and policy cast greater focus toward school lunch, the detail and frequency with which she spoke of parents was radically different. Brenda also saw the PTA in specific ways: "PTA, you get a snap shot of a particular group of people. We don't get the whole range of diversity that's represented in our district at PTA meetings."

17 Countless examples of this emerged. Parents had called to complain about three flat-screen TVs that televise news during the lunch period, saying, "Kids are bombarded with media, do they have to be in school too?" In another case, which I learned of from one of the lunchroom monitors, a student had discovered that the milk had expired, kids texted their parents, and within an hour, several phone calls had been made.

18 According to U.S. Census statistics, less than 3 percent of families are below the poverty line within the school district.

19 The website of the town where Washington is located states that parents had successfully obtained the town's school system's separation from the larger county school district in an effort to establish "a highly acclaimed school system." With less than five thousand households, it is a small hamlet. The community has a feel of being tightly knit, though in all likelihood that feeling is derived more from the shared commitment to a particular lifestyle choice than to strong social bonds.

20 The subject of the trays also emerged as an issue at Thurgood for Brenda. "We are working toward more environmentally responsible trays but the ones we tested were not engineered well." They collapsed or melted, Brenda told me, when the food was placed on them because of temperature requirements. She explained to me that while she'd like to spend the twelve cents on better trays, she would continue to use the three-cent polystyrene trays and use that "other eight and half cents for fruits and vegetable or whole grain. So I tell parents those are the deci-

sions you have to make. I would rather pour that money back into food for these kids, you know healthier foods or better-tasting foods for them."

21 The hyperinvolvement of parents was a point every single adult I spoke to at the school mentioned. Joe, who provided security and monitored the lunchroom for the school, told me on one occasion that the parents were the worst: "They text their kids. But these are good kids, good school, a big focus on education—that's the worst thing—kids don't cheat nothing." He said the "parents are a problem—really involved but won't believe their kids could do some of the things they do—even if you have footage, 'That's not my son,'" he said. Later Mr. Hudson, another staff person, told me that kids text parents if something is wrong at school.

22 Sociologist Peggy Nelson (2011), in her book *Parenting out of Control,* found in her interviews with professional, upper-middle-class parents that the parent-child communication was frequent and intensive. See also Armstrong and Hamilton, 2013; Lareau, 2000; Lareau, 2003; Pugh, 2009.

23 See also Newman, 1999.

24 1992: 152.

25 Johnston, Szabo, and Rodney, 2011.

26 1984: 77.

27 Though much has changed since 2010 in the commercial food landscape. Many of these food items are much more widely available.

28 Pirate's Booty, a favorite among professional middle-class parents into "healthy snacks," is too expensive, I learned later from Dan, who didn't stock any items that would cost more than $1.25.

29 Cairns, Johnston, and McKendrick, 2013.

30 What sort of assumptions do schools make about homes? Both Dan and Brenda assumed that kids were largely rearing themselves. I think we need to be cautious in making those claims.

31 See PR Newswire, "Consumer Snacking Habits and Impulse Foods Market Trends Reviewed to Help Effectively Target New Consumer Groups and Behaviors," www.prnewswire.com (downloaded Sept. 18, 2012).

32 Johnston and Baumann, 2015: 41.

33 Bourdieu, 1984: 190.

34 I am referring to openly expressed food complaints. I was not privy to food complaints outside the cafeteria.

35 I am borrowing the conceptual frame Johnston and Bauman (2015) develop between democracy and distinction to understand the gourmet food landscape.

36 I told her I usually ate what I saw the bulk of the kids eating, and she wished me luck and walked back to her table, where she collected her things and exited the room.

37 1984: 84.

38 I saw few kids at Thurgood wearing college t-shirts. Instead, kids wore high school t-shirts with school colors.

39 This was not seen at Thurgood.

40 Amy Wilkins's (2008) excellent analysis of the Goth scene also identifies the theme of limited liability for upper-middle-class kids, who can broker in a type of marginalized cool without forfeiting later mobility that other forms of youth rebellion threaten.

41 One can easily see how commercial foods are what Allison Pugh (2009) has called "scrip," which she recognizes as highly "salient to peer culture" (7). The value of outside commercial foods was especially apparent at Washington. At Thurgood, as I already noted, very little outside food was present in the cafeteria. The food made in the culinary arts classroom, however, was coveted by students. Their classroom adjoined the kitchen and lunchroom. When students were released from the class, they often came through the cafeteria and in many cases were met by small huddles of students interested in what they had prepared that day and hoping for a taste, which in most cases they were denied.

42 And in this sense, outside food also placed a burden on the holder of the food, since the expectation often was that the food would be shared. Gender over-whelmingly patterned how these exchanges unfolded. In the case where a request of food was made but rejected, boys were more likely to persist in their requests, hopeful that eventually the other would submit and forsake the item in question. During one lunch, I observed a group of six Washington boys, all freshmen, with traces of acne and braces, eating their lunch together. One of the boys, tall and lanky, pulled out a pack of gum and another boy immediately perked up, reach-ing his hand out before the boy had even opened the container. He pulled the container back from the grabbing boy and then pulled out what looked like a thin sliver of gum, wrapped in black tinfoil, and handed it to the boy. Just then, one of the other boys chimed in, "Split it with me." This he repeated two more times be-fore the boy relented and handed him over his half, which he quickly tossed into his mouth, despite not having finished his sandwich. I did not observe a single instance of a girl persisting in this manner. A request would be made, and if it was rejected, the matter was closed.

43 I also observed a handful of mini–birthday parties for girls by girls at Thurgood.

44 See for instance, Hey, 1997; Eder, Evans, and Parker, 1995.

45 There was some exception to this rule. I observed at Thurgood attempts made by girls to get boys to share food from their school lunch trays, which was almost always refused. The symbolic weight of the gesture is meaningful in terms of gendered status relations between boys and girls, a point I return to in chapter 5.

46 1971: 195.

47 Take as another example the sharing of a water bottle. Is a person permitted to place his lips to the rim of another young person's water bottle, or is he instead obligated to hold the bottle an inch from his lips as water carefully pours into his mouth? I came to appreciate that the sharing of a water bottle communicates the strength of a relationship and provides evidence of intimate ties between two people. It is as much an expression of social convention as of concerns for health

and the spread of germs. The only cases where lips were permitted to touch the rim of another's bottle were those of boyfriend and girlfriend and thus were bound up with public norms about heterosexual coupling. I did observe kids jokingly pretend to transgress this rule, almost putting their lips to the bottle and retreating only in the last second. We might think about these exchanges as rituals of avoidance, to borrow again from Goffman, which implies a commitment to not swap spit, and thereby enables young people to honor their obligation to share with friends, without having to cross boundaries of "personal territories" publicly, since that might be taken as evidence of romantic or sexually intimate ties. This was especially important for the sharing that occurred between guys and girls since it eliminated any confusion as to the nature of their relationship. I never observed boys sharing water bottles with other boys.

48 Douglas, 1966.

49 I also observed students at Washington share with the good-natured intent to broaden someone's cultural world. For example, I once observed three boys at a table with a small tray of California rolls in front of them. One boy, eyeing the California roll, asked the other boy what he was supposed to do and he showed by example, opening a soy sauce pouch and trickling it over the Nori, remarking that he liked the avocado in it. The other boy took a bite and let it be known with a gesture of his face that he did not care for it. "I love it," the other boy declared.

50 There are not enough cases to conclude that this is about masculine friendship norms, but I raise here the possibility that these tussles are more numerous among boys. Most disputes I observed around food gifting were between boys.

51 Think about how college students complain about the cost of books (which are admittedly expensive), even as they are willing to spend significant money on iPhones and other high-value consumables. These are ultimately questions of value.

52 For very good discussion on the tensions among class, schooling, and democratic commitments, see Khan 2012 and Reay et al. 2008.

CHAPTER 5. I'M LOVIN' IT

1 Hip-hop has long been a cultural site allowing for organically arising artistic creation by youth, on the one hand, but has been aggressively coopted by commercial markets, facilitating widespread appeal of the musical form among youth, on the other.

2 1990. See also Warikoo, 2013, for a discussion of the global youth currency hip-hop holds.

3 2010: 132.

4 Bennett, 2003: Brumberg, 1997; Harris, 2004; Marshall, 2010; McRobbie, 1991, 1993, Miles, 2000; Paterson, 2006.

5 See, for example, Michael Moss's (2013) *Salt, Sugar, Fat: How Food Giants Hooked Us.*

6 See Ritzer, 2005, and Schlosser, 2001, for example, for discussion of the standardized dimension of fast-food production and consumption. Fantasia (1995) situates fast food simultaneously in symbolic and material realms, arguing that "we can discern ever more clearly the material dimensions of culture and the non-material dimensions of goods" (201) when full attention is given to the place of context and meaning in the consumption of goods. Fantasia's aim is to move beyond a framework of "foodways" by considering "fast food outlets as distinctive places" that exist within a symbolic economy. "What kind of thing is the fast-food phenomenon in France?" Fantasia asks (202) as he goes on to show the importance of understanding the situationally specific repertoires of meaning of the goods and the space of McDonald's that adolescent consumers carried. In this case, national context and national identity meaningfully patterned meaning-making process, that is, how youth apprehended McDonald's as a social object.

7 Yan, 2005.

8 A fact that is sometimes overlooked in our discussions of childhood obesity.

9 See Palladino, 1997.

10 1989.

11 The postschool "rush" falls within what anthropologists of food typically regard as an unstructured food event. While the event is recurring, it tends to be spontaneous, loosely bound, and arising informally. The ritual aspects includes queuing behavior, a standard transcript for ordering ("Give me a number 2, Big Mac, small fries"), and the relatively uniform removal and discarding of unwanted materials as part of exiting procedures. McDonald's demands its own expertise or communicative competence in that one needs to know how to order. Whereas I stumble, these kids are experts, efficient in ordering. This is part of the appeal of the standardized fare McDonald's peddles.

12 The affective gains of moments serve to orient youth to the setting. These gains provide loose outline for the construction of meaning and serve as guide for action within a consumer realm, what Goffman in his seminal *Frame Analysis* (1974) referred to as "keying." Keying, for Goffman, is "a process of transcription" (44) "by which a given activity, already meaningful in terms of some primary framework, is transformed into something patterned on this activity but seen by the participants to be something quite else" (43–44). (See Goffman 1963, 1967, 1971, 1974, 1983.) For a more detailed elaboration of this line of argument see Best, 2014.

13 See also Halkier and Jensen, 2011.

14 See, for example, Marshall, 2010.

15 See also Swidler, 1986.

16 Goffman, 1974, 1971.

17 I have omitted the citation because to do so would identify the town.

18 As Austin et al. (2005) have reported.

19 It is probably noteworthy that most objections (though not all) to McDonald's were lodged by upper-middle-class girls, which reflects the entanglements of class and gender.

20 Though, on the other hand, class resources enable greater choice.

21 It is less common today to be denied service at the counter, but fast-food restaurants often opt out of poor markets in low-income communities, foreclosing
consumer options for the poor and thus perpetuating a form of exclusion.

22 Much like other schools, Hampton High is a space of racial sorting. As one white
student remarked to me in an interview, unless a student is in AP (advanced
placement) classes, life at Hampton High is like "ghetto immersion." This racial
arrangement has some relevance for understanding the racial geography of the
Hampton McDonald's. And in this sense a racial segmentation similar to Thurgood's may be in play in this commercial space.

23 I suspect, however, that participation in football and basketball helps to pattern
this arrangement.

24 Competing racial realities exist alongside each other at this McDonald's. While
participants are largely black, a different transcript of race and place is communicated through images that hang on the walls—images of McDonald's "nostalgic"
past—a racial past where happy, blonde-headed, freckle-faced teens occupied a
place on both sides of the counter—a boy with two thumbs up, another teenage
boy in starched white pants and shirt and crisp white hat who serves fifteen-
cent hamburgers and ten-cent Orangeade. Today, the workers are largely brown,
female, and adult—most appearing to be South Asian. Adult immigrant workers are something I have come to expect. Immigrant adult workers increasingly
have been regarded as more reliable and desirable than teen labor, as both Robin
Leidner (1993) in *Fast Food, Fast Talk: Service Work and the Routinization of
Everyday Life* and Katherine Newman (2000) in her ethnography on low-income
urban service workers, *No Shame in My Game*, also note.

25 As I discussed in chapter 1, young people's increasingly busy schedules intervene in family food provisioning. Young people's consumption of fast food is
often shaped by their after-school schedule of extracurricular activities, which
because of the high number of activities sponsored by school, are staggered.
There is not enough room for all sports teams, for example, to practice directly
after school. For some kids, sports practice doesn't occur until 5:00 in the
afternoon. For kids who live close to school or have a car or a parent available
to drive them, they can go home, work on their homework, and then return for
practice. But other kids, who rely exclusively on the school bus system, are stuck
at school.

26 Importantly, while the student base tends to be Anglo, the food workers are all
young and brown—again, none are teens. Here an ethno-racial link to food is
demonstrated through food service, not food consumption. The food's claim of
ethnic authenticity is supported by the brown workers.

27 Bell and Valentine, 1997; Best, 2000; Best, 2006; Bugge, 2011; Cross, 2004; Steinberg and Kincheloe, 1997; McRobbie, 1991; Miles, 2000; Thornton, 1994, 1995.

28 See also Harrison and Morgan, 2005, for a discussion of the formation of a teen interactional order in commercial food space in and against an adult interactional order.

29 Bell and Valentine, 1997; Counihan and Kaplan, 1998; DeVault, 1991: Douglas, 1972, 1966; Geertz, 1973; Greenbaum, 2012: Halkier and Jensen, 2011; Hochschild, 1997; Mintz, 1986. Most would also agree there is a deep relational character to food as a consumer good (Bordo, 1993; Eberstadt, 2009).

30 Illouz, 2009: 388.

31 2009: 388. Other actors, both situational and institutional, beside McDonald's, for instance, can and do serve as arbiters of the meaning of the food object.

32 Goffman, 1977: 324.

33 1995.

34 2009: 7.

35 Pugh, 2009: 81. Yet, this was not the case at Chipotle, where any exchange of money occurred underground and was not part of a publicly managed terrain. In settings that don't bear a youth imprint, this money talk would be seen as a breach of conduct.

36 Miller, 2001: 111.

37 In all my observations, I saw one instance of a kid using a bank card.

38 A point made by one of the reviewers.

39 Goffman, 1967.

40 This is well in line with Bourdieu's (1984) ideas about formalism and displays of the body as formed and patterned through class habitus, though I suggest here that much more important to understanding patterns of action is the structure of the situation.

41 See Zelizer, 1985, for a discussion of sacralization. In chapter 3, I argued that teenagers' actions at Washington reflected the cultural logic of the professional middle class in terms of their general engagements with food, their evaluation of it, and their requests for modification. But the analysis here suggests that the system of disposition formulated by Bourdieu applies less neatly to teenagers when in youth cultural scenes. It is the case that "aesthetic categories" and their cultural logic privileged by teens are sometimes intended to be understood by youth alone, to mark the distinction between youth and adults, and, thus, are not always reflecting a set of class arrangements.

42 1984: 90.

43 1967: 3.

44 1997: 119.

45 See Randall Collins, 2004, for a discussion of interactional rituals

46 For example, the Center for Science in the Public Interest, a group that has worked ardently to hold regulatory bodies and corporations accountable to children's health, often adopts a framework that eclipses youth agency and elides recognition of the symbolic work youth undertake in these commercial settings.

47 Collins, 2004: 37.

48 I have focused on the affective gains and emotional charge of the cultural scene. As sociologist Eva Illouz (2009) argues, "[E]motion compels us to action."

49 Paying greater attention to situations and their structure should not be at the expense of continued attention to structures, as Goffman himself argued (see 1967, 1971). Con-

tinued attention to the structural dimension of markets and consumer practices is indeed important. One reason why this is the case is that the situations in which youth consume do in fact render invisible the relations of commodity exchange in which youth are engaged, displacing a focus on markets and consumption for youth themselves. We certainly should not ignore the fact that young people are spending money on food derived from an industrial agricultural complex, that a large chunk of their time is spent in commercial settings, that the market does restratify youth groups, and that there are tangible health outcomes for youth. But, we should proceed with attention to situations and their structure, along with structures themselves.

CONCLUSION

1 Today, the Woolworth's counter, which is permanently placed on exhibit at the National Museum of American History, is enshrined in our collective memory of the power of the people and their struggle for freedom to end an unjust system of racial segregation and persecution.

2 Levine, 2008.

3 This thinking is in line with Eviatar Zerubavel's (1984) conception of social cognition, as discussed in *The Fine Line.*

4 Thornton, 1995.

5 Bell and Valentine, 1997; Bugge, 2011.

6 "The meaning of the object," as Erving Goffman explained decades ago, then, "is generated through its use" (1974: 39). "Objects can be modified but not totally recreated" because "the meaning of an object is a product of social definition. . . . I do not mean to imply that no stable meaning is built socially into artifacts, merely that circumstances can enforce an additional meaning" (39).

7 They refuse to refuse that which belongs to the realm of the vulgar, a behavioral expectation largely associated with middle-class adulthood and the feminine. This is in line with Bourdieu's thinking on youth as a period for the bourgeoisie when class tastes are temporarily suspended.

8 Bourdieu, 1984: 477.

9 2001: 21.

10 Hochschild, 1997.

11 Guthman (2009) attributes this to the rise of neoliberal forms of governance. "Neoliberal governmentality is also characterized by efforts to shift caring responsibilities from public spheres (welfare) to personal spheres (self-help). . . . If neoliberalism as a project is concerned with creating subjects capable of making nominally free choices . . . it stands to reason that the good neo-liberal subject would strive for fitness, a marker of capability" (1116). In this discursive context, thin bodies come to be associated with discipline, personal responsibility, and self-control, and fat bodies come to signify the absence of those virtues, and anxiety about them intensifies.

12 A 2009 USDA report found that children who participated in NSLP had reduced sugar-beverage intake and fewer calories from low-nutrient, energy-dense foods in school. See Gleason et al., 2009.

13 Alexander (2006) in his seminal *Civil Sphere* discusses this in terms of generalized versus particularistic concerns.

14 Binkley, 2010: 653.

15 Giddens (1991) attributes this to a series of institutional transformations, which include a separation of time and space, new modes of specialized technical knowledge, globalization, and disembedding of local existence resulting from the emergence of abstract systems of money economy and experts.

16 See Ulrich Beck's (1992) arguments about risk society, risk distribution, and the boomerang effect as fundamental consequence of modernization.

17 2010: 650.

18 2010: 652.

19 See Tom Hamburger, "Boardroom Tries to Reach into Lunchroom," *Washington Post*, May 30, 2014, A1, A4.

20 While schools have been subject to intensifying critique, substantial research, for example, has shown that children are more likely to gain weight in the summer months, a period when the bulk of their time is spent outside of school, not in it. Summer months, especially for the lower-income kids, without a full roster of structured camp activity, are months marked by increased down time, a period of less adult supervision.

21 2003: 39.

22 2009.

23 2013: 139.

24 2013: 153–54.

25 Rollins et al., 2014.

26 The need to appreciate the meaning particular food holds for different groups was argued by the famous anthropologist Margaret Mead to the federal government in the 1940s in her work with the USDA. See documents in the 2012 National Archives exhibit, "What's Cooking, Uncle Sam?" at http://www.archives.gov.

27 A colleague of mine relayed a story to me as I was concluding data collection for this project and exiting the field. She had recently attended a council meeting for her ward. School food was one of the agenda items, and some high school students had prepared remarks to present to the council, providing feedback on how the D.C. Healthy School Act was being implemented in their respective schools. The teens presented their case, acknowledging the significant improvements in the healthy offerings in school but also asking for more options and the expansion of food choices. This was heard by the responding council member incorrectly as a complaint about the shortage of healthy food options, suggesting that he was unable to hear anything outside the health frame.

METHODS APPENDIX

1 Geertz, 1973: 17.

2 1998: 85.

3 1998: 96–97.

4 D. Smith (1999), *Writing the Social: Critique, Theory, and Investigations* (Toronto: University of Toronto Press); D. Smith (1990), *Texts, Facts, and Femininity: Exploring the Relations of Ruling* (New York: Routledge); D. Smith (1990), *The Conceptual Practices of Power: A Feminist Sociology of Knowledge* (Boston: Northeastern University Press); D. Smith (1987), *The Everyday World as Problematic: A Feminist Method* (Boston: Northeastern University Press).

5 1973: 10.

6 Best, 2007.

7 See Best, 2000, 2006, 2007.

8 Fieldnotes, the written representational accounts of the observed activity, should be descriptively rich, with the explicit aim to capture scenes on a page in vivid detail. Judgments are to be withheld and analysis should be postponed until there is a reasonable collection of materials from which to draw. Close jottings (note taking) were recorded in the field in a small notebook. After I left the field, jottings were developed into fieldnotes. As a general rule of thumb, for every hour spent observing, two hours were spent writing fieldnotes. The end product was several sets of deeply detailed descriptions of action as it unfolded contemporaneously.

9 1963: 4.

10 Glaser and Strauss, 1967.

11 Geertz, 1973: 27.

12 1959.

13 Small, 2009.

14 In defining "middle income," I exclude the income groups in the bottom 20 percent and top 20 percent of the U.S. population.

15 D.C. Hunger Solutions reports that "[o]f the city's 43 full-service grocery stores, only four are in Ward 7, and three in Ward 8. By contrast, Ward 3—the highest-income Ward—has eleven full-service stores." See "When Healthy Food Is Out of Reach: An Analysis of the Grocery Gap in the District of Columbia 2010." See also "Facts on Hunger in DC," http://www.dchunger.org.

16 I involved two graduate students, Katie Kerstetter and J. L. Johnson, in data collection for the evaluation of these programs; one student was funded by a Kaiser Permanente HEAL grant.

REFERENCES

Adamick, K. 2012. *Lunch Money: Serving Healthy School Food in a Sick Economy*. New York: Food Systems Solutions.

Adler, P., and P. Adler. 1998. *Peer Power*. New Brunswick, NJ: Rutgers University Press.

Adler, P., and P. Adler. 1987. *Membership Roles in Field Research*. Newbury Park, CA: Sage.

Adler, Thomas. 1981. "Making Pancakes on Sunday: The Male Cook in Family Tradition." *Western Folklore* 40.1: 45–54.

Alexander, J. 2006. *The Civil Sphere*. Oxford: Oxford University Press.

Allen, P., and J. Guthman. 2006. "From 'Old School' to 'Farm-to-School': Neoliberalization from the Ground Up." *Agriculture and Human Values* 23: 401–15.

Anyon, J. 1997. *Ghetto Schooling: A Political Economy of Urban Educational Reform*. New York: Teacher's College Press, Columbia University.

Appadurai, A. (ed.). 1986. *The Social Life of Things: Commodities in Cultural Perspective*. New York: Cambridge University Press.

Apple, M. W., and L. Weis. 1983. *Ideology and Practice in Schooling*. Philadelphia: Temple University Press.

Armstrong, E., and L. Hamilton. 2013. *Paying the Party: How College Maintains Inequality*. Cambridge, MA: Harvard University Press.

Austin, S. B., S. Melly, B. Sanchez, A. Patel, S. Buka, and S. Gortmaker. 2005. "Clustering of Fast-Food Restaurant around Schools: A Novel Application of Spatial Statistics to the Study of Food Environments." *American Journal of Public Health* 95.9: 1575–81.

Barthes, R. 1997. "Toward a Psychosociology of Contemporary Food Consumption." *Food and Culture: A Reader*. 2nd ed. Eds. Carole Counihan and Penny Van Esterik. New York: Routledge.

Bauman, Z. 2001. *The Individualized Society*. London: Polity.

Bauman, Z. 2000. *Liquid Modernity*. Cambridge: Polity.

Baylis, J., and S. Wang. 2011. "Racism on Aisle Two: A Survey of Federal and State Antidiscrimination Public Accommodation Laws." *William and Mary Policy Review*, 288–311.

Beardsworth, A., and T. Keil. 1997. *Sociology on the Menu: An Invitation to the Study of Food and Society*. New York: Routledge.

Beck, U. 1992. *Risk Society: Towards a New Modernity*. New Delhi: Sage. (Translated from the German edition published by Risikogesellschaft in 1986.)

Belasco, W. 2008. *Food: The Key Concepts*. New York: Berg.

Bell, D., and G. Valentine (eds.). 1997. *Consuming Geographies: We Are Where We Eat*. New York: Routledge.

Bellah, R. N., R. Madsen, W. Sullivan, A. Swidler, and S. M. Tipton. 1985. *Habits of the Heart: Individualism and Commitment in American Life*. Berkeley: University of California Press.

Bennett, A. 2003. "Subcultures or Neo-tribes? Rethinking the Relationship between Youth, Style, and Musical Taste." In *The Consumption Reader*. Eds. D. B. Clarke, M. Doel, and K. L. Housiaux. London: Routledge.

Bennett, A., and K. Kahn-Harris (eds.) 2004. *After Subculture: Critical Studies in Contemporary Youth Culture*. London: Palgrave-Macmillan.

Beresin, A. 2010. *Recess Battles: Playing, Fighting, and Storytelling*. Jackson: University Press of Mississippi.

Berger, P., and T. Luckmann. 1966. *The Social Construction of Reality: A Treatise in the Sociology of Knowledge*. New York: Doubleday.

Berk, L. 2005. "Why Parenting Matters." In *Childhood Lost: How American Culture Is Failing Our Kids*. Ed. Sharna Olfman. Westport, CT: Praeger.

Besen-Cassino, Y. 2014. *Consuming Work: Youth Labor in America*. Philadelphia, PA: Temple University Press.

Best, A. L. 2014. "Youth Consumers and the Fast-Food Market: The Emotional Landscape of Micro-Encounters, Situations as Guide for Action." *Food, Culture, and Society: An International Journal of Interdisciplinary Research* 18.2: 283–300.

Best, A. 2008. "Teen Driving as Public Drama: Statistics, Risk, and the Social Construction of Youth as a Public Problem." *Journal of Youth Studies* 11.6: 651–71.

Best, A. 2007. *Representing Youth: Methodological Issues in Critical Youth Studies*. New York: NYU Press.

Best, A. 2006. *Fast Cars, Cool Rides: The Accelerating World of Youth and Their Cars*. New York: NYU Press.

Best, A. 2000. *Prom Night: Youth, Schools, and Popular Culture*. New York: Routledge.

Best, J. 2001. *Damned Lies and Statistics: Untangling Numbers from the Media, Politicians, and Activists*. Berkeley: University of California Press.

Bettie, J. 2003. *Women without Class: Girls, Race, and Identity*. Berkeley: University of California Press.

Bianchi, S., J. Robinson, and M. Milkie. 2007. *Changing Rhythms of Family Life*. New York: Russell Sage Foundation.

Biltekoff, C. 2013. *Eating Right in America: The Cultural Politics of Food and Health*. Durham, NC: Duke University Press.

Binkley, S. 2010. "Cultural Movements and the Sociology of Culture: The Case of Political Consumerism." In *Sociology of Culture: A Handbook*. Eds. L. Grindstaff, J. Hall, and M. Lo. New York: Routledge

Boero, N. 2012. *Killer Fat: Media, Medicine, and Morals in the American "Obesity Epidemic."* New Brunswick, NJ: Rutgers University Press.

Boero, N. 2009. "Fat Kids, Working Moms, and the 'Epidemic of Obesity': Race, Class, and Mother Blame." In *The Fat Studies Reader*. Eds. E. Rothblum and S. Solovay. New York: NYU Press.

Bordo, S. 1993. *Unbearable Weight: Feminism, Western Culture, and the Body*. Berkeley: University of California Press.

Bourdieu, P. 1984. *Distinction: A Social Critique of the Judgment of Taste*. Cambridge, MA: Harvard University Press.

Brembeck, H. 2009. "Children's Becoming in Frontiering Foodscapes." *Children, Food, and Identity in Everyday Life*. Eds. A. James, A. Trine Kjirholt, and V. Tingstad. New York: Palgrave Macmillan.

Brown, L. M. 1998. *Raising Their Voices: The Politics of Girls' Anger*. Cambridge, MA: Harvard University Press.

Brumberg, J. J. 1997. "The Appetite as Voice." *Food and Culture: A Reader*. 2nd ed. Eds. C. Counihan and P. Van Esterik. New York: Routledge.

Brumberg, J. J. 1997. *The Body Project: An Intimate History of American Girls*. New York: Random House.

Brumberg, J. J. 1988. *Fasting Girls: The Emergence of Anorexia Nervosa as a Modern Disease*. Cambridge, MA: Harvard University Press.

Bugge, A. B. 2011. "Lovin' It? A Study of Youth and the Culture of Fast-Food." *Food, Culture, and Society*. 14.11: 71–89.

Cairns, K., J. Johnston, and N. McKendrick. 2013. "Feeding the 'Organic Child': Mothering through Ethical Consumption." *Journal of Consumer Culture* 13.2: 97–118.

Campos, P. 2004. *The Obesity Myth: Why America's Obsession with Weight Is Hazardous to Your Health*. New York: Gotham.

Campos, P., A. Saguy, P. Ernsberger, E. Oliver, and G. Gaesser. 2006. "The Epidemiology of Overweight and Obesity: Public Health Crisis or Moral Panic?" *International Journal of Epidemiology* 35.1: 55–60.

Carter, P. 2005. *Keepin' It Real: School Success beyond Black and White*. Oxford: Oxford University Press.

Carter, P. 2003. "'Black' Cultural Capital, Status Positioning, and Schooling Conflicts for Low-Income African American Youth." *Social Problems* 50.1: 136–55.

Cherlin, A. 2009. *The Marriage Go-Around: The State of Marriage and Family in America Today*. New York: Random House.

Chin, E. 2001. "Feminist Theory and the Ethnography of Children's Worlds: Barbie in New Haven, Connecticut." In *Children and Anthropology: Perspectives for the 21st Century*. Ed. H. Schwartzman. Westport, CT: Bergin and Garvey.

Chin, E. 2001. *Purchasing Power: Black Kids and American Consumer Culture*. Minneapolis: University of Minnesota Press.

Christensen, P., and A. James (eds.). 2000. *Research with Children: Perspectives and Practices*. London: Falmer.

Cinotto, S. 2006. "'Everyone Would Be around the Table': American Family Mealtimes in Historical Perspective, 1850–1960." *New Directions for Child and Adolescent Development*, no. 111: 17–34.

Clark, H. R., E. Goyder, P. Bissell, L. Blank, and J. Peters. "How Do Parents' Child-Feeding Behaviours Influence Child Weight? Implications for Childhood Obesity Policy." *Journal of Public Health* 29.2: 131–42.

Clay, A. 2012. *The Hip-Hop Generation Fights Back: Youth, Activism, and Post–Civil Rights Politics*. New York: NYU Press.

Colgrove, J., G. Markowitz, and D. Rosner (eds.). 2008. *The Contested Boundaries of American Health*. New Brunswick, NJ: Rutgers University Press.

Collins, R. 2004. *Interaction Ritual Chains*. Princeton, NJ: Princeton University Press.

Conley, D. 2009. *Elsewhere, U.S.A.: How We Got from the Company Man, Family Dinner, and the Affluent Society to the Home Office, Blackberry Moms, and Economic Anxiety*. New York: Vintage.

Connolly, P. 1998. *Racism, Gender Identities, and Young Children: Social Relations in a Multi-Ethnic, Inner-City Primary School*. London: Routledge.

Cook, D. 2009. "Children's Subjectivities and Commercial Meaning: The Delicate Battle Mothers Wage When Feeding Their Children." *Children, Food, and Identity in Everyday Life*. Eds. A. James, A. Trine Kjirholt, and V. Tingstad. New York: Palgrave Macmillan.

Cook, D. 2004. *The Commodification of Childhood: The Children's Clothing Industry and the Rise of the Child Consumer*. Durham, NC: Duke University Press.

Coontz, S. 1992. *The Way We Never Were: American Families and the Nostalgia Trap*. New York: Basic Books.

Corsaro, W. 2012. "Interpretive Reproduction in Children's Play." *American Journal of Play* 4.4: 488–504.

Corsaro, W. 2003. *We're Friends Right? Inside Kids' Culture*. Washington, DC: Joseph Henry Press.

Counihan, C. (ed.). 2002. *Food in the U.S.A.: A Reader*. New York: Routledge.

Counihan, C., and S. Kaplan (eds.). 1998. *Food and Gender: Identity and Power*. Australia: Harwood Academic Publishers.

Counihan, C., and P. Van Esterik (eds.). 1997. *Food and Culture: A Reader*. 2nd ed. New York: Routledge.

Covic, T., L. Roufeil, and S. Dziurawiec. 2007. "Community Beliefs about Childhood Obesity: Its Causes, Consequences, and Potential Solutions." *Journal of Public Health* 29.2: 123–31.

Cross, G. 2004. "Gremlin Child: How the Cute Became the Cool." In *The Cute and the Cool: Wondrous Innocence and Modern American Children's Culture*. Oxford: Oxford University Press.

De Certeau, M. 1984. *The Practice of Everyday Life*: Berkeley: University of California Press.

De Garine, I., and N. Pollock (eds.). 1995. *Social Aspects of Obesity*. Australia: Gordon and Breach.

DeVault, M. 1991. *Feeding the Family: The Social Organization of Caring as Gendered Work*. Chicago: University of Chicago Press.

Dolphijn, R. 2004. *Foodscapes: Toward a Deleuzian Ethics of Consumption*. Delft: Eburon Press.

Douglas, M. 1973. *Food in the Social Order: Mary Douglas, Collected Works*. New York: Routledge.

Douglas, M. 1972. "Deciphering a Meal." *Daedalus* 101: 61–81.

Douglas, M. 1966. *Purity and Danger: An Analysis of Concepts of Pollution and Purity*. London: Routledge & Kegan Paul.

Eberstadt, M. 2009. "Is Food the New Sex? A Curious Moral Reversal." *Policy Review* 153 (February/March). http://www.hoover.org.

Eckert, P. 1989. *Jocks and Burnouts: Social Categories and Identity in High School*. New York: Teacher's College Press, Columbia University.

Eder, D., C. Evans, and S. Parker. 1995. *School Talk: Gender and Adolescent Culture*. New Brunswick, NJ: Rutgers University Press.

Emerson, R. M., R. I. Fretz, and L. Shaw. 1995. *Writing Ethnographic Fieldnotes*. Chicago: University of Chicago Press.

Epstein, J. (ed.). 2001. *Youth Culture: Identity in a Postmodern World*. Oxford: Blackwell.

Erikson, E. 1968. *Identity: Youth and Crisis*. New York: Norton.

Etzioni, A., and J. Bloom (eds.). 2004. *We Are What We Celebrate: Understanding Holidays and Rituals*. New York: NYU Press.

Evans, M., and E. Lee. 2002. *Real Bodies: A Sociological Introduction* New York: Palgrave Macmillan.

Fantasia, R. 1995. "Fast-Food in France." *Theory and Society* 24.2: 201–43.

Ferguson, A. 2001. *Bad Boys: Public Schools in the Making of Black Masculinity*. Ann Arbor: University of Michigan Press.

Fitzpatrick, K., and M. LaGory. 2000. *Unhealthy Places: The Ecology of Risk in the Urban Landscape*. New York: Routledge.

Foley, D. 2005. "Performance Theory and Critical Ethnography: Studying Chicano and Mesquaki Youth." In *Performance Theories in Education: Power, Pedagogy, and the Politics of Identity*. Eds. B. Alexander, G. Anderson, and B. Gallegos. Mahwah, NJ: Erlbaum.

Furlong, A. (ed.). 2007. *Handbook of Youth and Young Adulthood: New Perspectives and Agendas*. New York: Routledge.

Furlong, A., and F. Cartmel. 1999. *Young People and Social Change: Individualization and Risk in Late Modernity*. Philadelphia: Open University Press.

Gaines, D. 1990. *Teenage Wasteland: Suburbia's Dead End Kids*. Chicago: University of Chicago Press.

Geertz, C. 1973. *The Interpretation of Cultures*: New York: Basic Books.

Germov, J., and L. Williams (eds.). 2008. *A Sociology of Food and Nutrition: The Social Appetite*. 3rd ed. Oxford: Oxford University Press.

Giddens, A. 1992. *The Transformation of Intimacy: Sexuality, Love, Eroticism in Modern Societies*. Palo Alto, CA: Stanford University Press.

Giddens, A. 1991. *Modernity and Self-Identity: Self and Society in the Late Modern Age.* Cambridge: Polity.

Gillis, J. 2004. "Gathering Together: Remembering Memory through Ritual." In *We Are What We Celebrate: Understanding Holidays and Rituals.* Eds. Amitai Etzioni and Jared Bloom. New York: NYU Press.

Glaser, B., and A. Strauss. 1967. *The Discovery of Grounded Theory: Strategies for Qualitative Research.* Chicago: Aldine.

Glassner, B. 2007. *The Gospel of Food: Why We Should Stop Worrying and Enjoy What We Eat.* New York: Harper.

Gleason, P., R. Briefel, A. Wilson, and A. H. Dodd. 2009. *School Meal Program Participation and Its Association with Dietary Patterns and Childhood Obesity.* Contractor and Cooperator Report, 55.Washington, DC: U.S. Department of Agriculture, Economic Research Service.

Goffman, E. 1983. "The Interaction Order: American Sociological Association, 1982 Presidential Address." *American Sociological Review* 48 (February): 1–17.

Goffman, E. 1974. *Frame Analysis: An Essay on the Organization of Experience.* New York: Harpers Colophon.

Goffman, E. 1971. *Relations in Public: Micro-Studies of the Public Order.* New York: Basic Books.

Goffman, E. 1967. *Interaction Ritual: Essays on Face-to-Face Behavior.* New York: Pantheon.

Goffman, E. 1963. *Behavior in Public Places: Notes on the Social Organization of Gatherings.* New York: Free Press.

Goffman, E. 1961. *Encounters: Two Studies in the Sociology of Interaction.* Indianapolis: Bobbs-Merrill.

Goffman, E. 1959. *Presentation of Self in Everyday Life.* New York: Doubleday Anchor.

Gong, Q., and P. Jackson. 2012. "Consuming Anxiety: Parenting Practices in China after the Infant Formula Scandal." *Food, Culture, and Society: An International Journal of Multidisciplinary Research* 15.4: 557–78.

Gosliner, W., K. Madsen, G. Woodward-Lopez, P. Crawford. 2011. "Would Students Prefer to Eat Healthier Foods at School?" *Journal of School Health* 81.3: 146–51.

Graebner, W. 1990. *Coming of Age in Buffalo: Youth and Authority in the Post War Era.* Philadelphia: Temple University Press.

Grasmuck, S. 2005. *Protecting Home: Class, Race, and Masculinity in Boys' Baseball.* New Brunswick, NJ: Rutgers University Press.

Gravlee, C. 2009. "How Race Becomes Biology: Embodiment of Social Inequality." *American Journal of Physical Anthropology* 139: 47–57.

Greenbaum, J. 2012. "Vegan Identity and the Quest for Authenticity." *Food, Culture, and Society* 15.1: 129–44.

Greenhalgh, S. 2015. *Fat-Talk Nation: The Human Costs of America's War on Fat.* New York: Cornell University Press.

Greenhalgh, S. 2012. "Weighty Subjects: The Bio-Politics of the War on Fat." *American Ethnologist* 39.3: 471–87.

Gregory, C. 2015. *Gifts and Commodities*. 2nd ed. Chicago: University of Chicago Press.

Griffin, C. 1993. "The Threat of Unstructured Free Time: Young People and Leisure in the 1980s." In *Representations of Youth: The Study of Youth and Adolescence in Britain and America*. London: Polity.

Gusfield, J. R. 1981. *The Culture of Public Problems: Drinking, Driving, and the Symbolic Order*. Chicago: University of Chicago Press.

Guthman, J. 2011. *Weighing In: Obesity, Food Justice, and the Limits of Capitalism*. California Studies in Food and Culture. Berkeley: University of California Press.

Guthman, J. 2009. "Teaching the Politics of Obesity: Insights into Neoliberal Embodiment and Contemporary Biopolitics." *Antipode* 41.5: 1110–33.

Halbwachs, M. 1992. *On Collective Memory* Chicago: University of Chicago Press.

Halkier, B., L. Holm, M. Domingues, P. Magguada, A. Neilsen, and L. Terragni. 2007. "Trusting, Complex, Quality Conscious, and Unprotected? Constructing the Food Consumer in Different European National Contexts." *Journal of Consumer Culture* 7.3: 379–402.

Halkier, B., and I. Jensen. 2011. "Methodological Challenges in Using Practice Theories in Consumption Research: Examples from a Study on Handling Nutritional Contestations of Food Consumption." *Journal of Consumer Culture*. 11.1: 101–23.

Hall, S., and T. Jefferson (eds.). 1975. *Resistance through Rituals*. London: Routledge.

Hamilton, J. 2013. "How Did Our Brains Evolve to Equate Food with Love?" *The Salt: What's On Your Plate*. http://www.npr.org.

Harrington Meyer, M. 2007. "Changing Marital Rates and Stagnant Social Security Policy." *Public Policy and Aging Report* 17.3 (Summer): 11–14. Washington, DC: National Academy on an Aging Society.

Harris, A. 2004. *Future Girl: Young Women in the Twenty-first Century*. New York: Routledge.

Harris, J., M. Schwartz, and K. Brownell. 2013. "Measuring Progression in Nutrition and Marketing to Children and Teens." Yale Rudd Center for Food Policy and Obesity.

Harris, J., M. Schwartz, and K. Brownell. 2010. "Evaluating Fast-Food Nutrition and Marketing to Youth." Fast-food F.A.C.T.S. Food Advertising to Children and Teens Score, Yale University Center for Food Policy and Obesity.

Harrison, T., and S. Morgan. 2005. "Hanging Out among Teenagers: Resistance, Gender, and Personal Relationships." In *Together Alone: Personal Relationships in Public Places*. Eds. C. Morrill, D. Snow, and C. White. Berkeley: University of California Press.

Harvey, D. 2007. *A Brief History of Neoliberalism*. Oxford: Oxford University Press.

Hayes-Conroy, J. 2009. "School Gardens and 'Actually Existing' Neoliberalism." *Humboldt Journal of Social Relations* 33.1/2: 64–96.

Hebdige, D. 1979. *Subculture: The Meaning of Style*. London: Routledge.

Hershman, J. 1998. "Massive Resistance Meets Its Match: The Emergence of a Pro–Public School Majority." In *The Moderates' Dilemma: Massive Resistance to School*

Desegregation in Virginia. Eds. Matthew Lassiter and Andrew Lewis. Charlottesville: University Press of Virginia, pp. 127–32.

Hewlett, S., and C. West. 2005. "The War against Parents." In *Childhood Lost: How American Culture Is Failing Our Kids*. Ed. S. Olfman. Westport, CT: Praeger.

Hey, V. 1997. *The Company She Keeps: An Ethnography of Girls' Friendships*. Philadelphia: Open University Press.

Hill, J. 2011. "Endangered Childhoods: How Consumerism Is Impacting Child/Youth Identity." *Media, Culture, and Society* 33.3: 347–62.

Hochschild, A. 2003. *The Commercialization of Intimate Life: Notes from Home and Work*. Berkeley: University of California Press.

Hochschild, A. 1997. *The Time Bind: When Work Becomes Home and Home Becomes Work*. New York: Metropolitan Books.

Hochschild, A. 1989. *The Second Shift: Working Parents and the Revolution at Home*. New York: Viking Penguin.

Illouz, E. 2009. "Emotions, Imagination, and Consumption: A New Research Agenda." *Journal of Consumer Culture* 9: 377–413.

Illouz, E. 2007. *Cold Intimacies*. Cambridge: Polity.

James, A., P. Curtis, and K. Ellis, 2009. "Negotiating Family, Negotiating Food: Children as Family Participants." In *Children, Food, and Family Life*. Eds. A. James, A. T. Kjorhold, and V. Tingstad. London: Palgrave.

Johnston, J., and S. Bauman. 2015. *Foodies: Democracy and Distinction in the Gourmet Foodscape*. New York: Routledge

Johnston, J., and S. Baumann. 2007. "Democracy versus Distinction: A Study of Omnivorousness in Gourmet Food Writing." *American Journal of Sociology* 113.1: 165–204.

Johnston, J., and K. Cairns. 2015. "Choosing Health, Embodied Neoliberalism, Postfeminism, and the 'Do Diet.'" *Theory and Society* 44: 153–75.

Johnston, J., M. Szabo, and A. Rodney. 2011. "Good Food, Good People: Understanding the Cultural Repertoire of Ethical Eating." *Journal of Consumer Culture* 11.3: 293–318.

Jones, N. 2010. *Between Good and Ghetto: African American Girls and Inner-City Violence*. New Brunswick, NJ: Rutgers University Press.

Kaplan, E. 2000. "Using Food as a Metaphor for Care: Middle School Kids Talk about Family, School, and Class Relationships." *Journal of Contemporary Ethnography* 29.4: 474–509.

Khan, S. 2012. *Privilege: The Making of an Adolescent Elite at St. Paul's School*. Princeton, NJ: Princeton University Press.

Kitsuse, J., and A. Cicourel. 1963. "A Note on the Official Uses of Statistics." *Social Problems* 11 (Fall): 131–39.

Klein, N. 2002. *No Logo*. New York: Picador.

Klinenberg, E. 2003. *Heat Wave: A Social Autopsy of Disaster in Chicago*. Chicago: University of Chicago Press.

Kotlowitz, A. 1991. *There Are No Children Here: The Story of Two Boys Growing Up in the Other America*. New York: Anchor Books.

Kozol, J. 1991. *Savage Inequalities*. New York: Crown.

Kunreuther, H. 1972. "Why the Poor May Pay More for Food: Theoretical and Empirical Evidence." In *Proceedings of the Third Annual Conference of the Association for Consumer Research*. Eds. Association for Consumer Research. Chicago: Association for Consumer Research, pp. 660–78.

Kuzawa, C., and E. Sweet. 2009. "Epigenetics and the Embodiment of Race: Developmental Origins of US Racial Disparities in Cardiovascular Health." *American Journal of Human Biology* 21: 2–15.

Lamont, M. 1992. *Money, Morals, and Manners: The Culture of the French and American Upper-Middle Class*. Chicago: University of Chicago Press.

Landsberg, A. 2004. *Prosthetic Memory: The Transformation of American Remembrance in the Age of Mass Culture*. New York: Columbia University Press.

Lareau, A. 2003. *Unequal Childhoods: Class, Race, and Family Life*. Berkeley: University of California Press.

Lareau, A. 2000. *Home Advantage: Social Class and Parental Intervention in Elementary School*. New York: Rowman & Littlefield.

Larson, R., K. Branscomb, and A. Wiley. 2006. "Forms and Functions of Family Mealtimes: Multidisciplinary Perspectives." *New Directions for Child and Adolescent Development* 2006.111: 115. Special Issue: Family Mealtime as a Context of Development and Socialization.

Lebesco, K. 2010. "Fat Panic and the New Morality." In *Against Health: How Health Became the New Morality*. Eds. J. Metzel and A. Kirkland. New York: NYU Press

Leidner, R. 1993. *Fast-Food, Fast Talk: Service Work and the Routinization of Everyday Life*. Berkeley: University of California Press.

Leonard, A. 2010. *The Story of Stuff: How Our Obsession with Stuff Is Trashing the Planet, Our Communities, and Our Health: A Vision for Change*. New York: Free Press.

Lesko, N. 2001. *Act Your Age: The Social Construction of Youth*. New York: Routledge.

Lesko, N. 1996. "Denaturalizing Adolescence: The Politics of Contemporary Representation." *Youth and Society* 28.2: 139–61.

Lesko, N. 1988. "The Curriculum of the Body: Lessons from a Catholic High School." In *Becoming Feminine: The Politics of Popular Culture*. Eds. Leslie G. Roman and Linda Christian-Smith. London: Falmer.

Levine, S. 2008. *School Lunch Politics: The Surprising History of America's Favorite Welfare Program*. Princeton, NJ: Princeton University Press.

Lobstein, T., L. Baur, and R. Uauy. 2004. "Obesity in Children and Young People: A Crisis in Public Health." *Obesity Reviews* 5.1: 4–85.

Lopez, N. 2003. *Hopeful Girls, Troubled Boys: Race and Gender Disparity in Urban Education*. New York: Routledge.

Lozado, E. 2005. "Globalized Childhood? Kentucky Fried Chicken in Beijing." In *The Cultural Politics of Food and Eating: A Reader*. Eds. J. Watson and M. Caldwell. Oxford: Blackwell.

Lupton, D. 1994. "Food Memory and Meaning: The Symbolic and Social Nature of Food Events." *Sociological Review* 42.4: 664–85.

Lupton, D. 1996. *Food, the Body, and the Self.* London: Sage.

Lynd, R., and H. Lynd.1929. *Middletown: A Study of American Culture.* New York: Harcourt, Brace, and World.

MacLeod, J. 1995. *Ain't No Making It: Aspirations and Attainment in a Low-Income Neighborhood.* Boulder, CO: Westview.

Maira, S. 2002. *Desis in the House: Indian American Youth Culture in New York City.* Philadelphia: Temple University Press.

Marshall, D. (ed.). 2010. *Understanding Children as Consumers.* Advanced Marketing Series. Thousand Oaks, CA: Sage.

Massengill, R. 2013. *Wal-Mart Wars: Moral Populism in the 21st Century New York*: NYU Press.

Marcus, G. 1998. "Ethnography in/of the World System: The Emergence of Multi-sited Ethnography." *Ethnography through Thick and Thin.* Princeton, NJ: Princeton University Press.

McDonald, K. 1999. *Struggle for Subjectivity: Identity, Action, and Youth Experience.* Cambridge: Cambridge University Press.

McRobbie, A. 1993. "Shut Up and Dance: Youth Culture and Changing Modes of Femininity." *Cultural Studies* 7: 406–25.

McRobbie, A. 1991. *Feminism and Youth Culture: From Jackie to Just Seventeen.* Boston: Unwin Hyman.

Mead, G. H. 1934. *Mind, Self, and Society: From the Standpoint of a Social Behaviorist.* Chicago: University of Chicago Press.

Metzl, J., and A. Kirkland (eds.). 2010. *Against Health: How Health Became the New Morality.* New York: NYU Press.

Miles, S. 2000. *Youth Lifestyles in a Changing World.* London: Open University Press.

Miller, D. 2001. "Alienable Gifts and Inalienable Commodities." In *The Empire of Things: Regimes of Value and Material Culture.* Ed. F. Myers. Santa Fe, NM: School of American Research Press.

Miller, J. 2008. *Getting Played: African American Girls; Urban Inequality and Gendered Violence.* New York: NYU Press.

Miller, J., and J. Deutsch. 2009. *Food Studies: An Introduction to Research Methods.* New York: Berg.

Milner, M. 2004. *Freaks, Geeks, and Cool Kids: American Teenagers, Schools, and the Culture of Consumption.* New York: Routledge.

Mintz, S. 1986. *Sweetness and Power: The Place of Sugar in Modern History.* New York: Penguin.

Moje, E. B., and C. Van Helden. 2005. "Doing Popular Culture: Troubling Discourses about Youth." In *Reconstructing the Adolescent: Sign, Symbol, Body.* Eds. J. Vadeboncoeur and L. Patel Stevens. New York: Peter Lang.

Moss, M. 2013. *Salt, Sugar, Fat: How the Food Giants Hooked Us.* New York: Random House.

Myers, F. (ed.). 2001. *The Empire of Things: Regimes of Value and Material Culture.* Santa Fe, NM: School of American Research Press.

Nayak, A., and M. J. Kehily. 2008. "Gender Relations in Late-Modernity: Young Femininities and the New Girl Order." *Gender, Youth, and Culture: Young Masculinities and Femininities.* New York: Palgrave Macmillan.

Nelson, M. 2011. *Parenting out of Control: Anxious Parents in Uncertain Times.* New York: NYU Press.

Nespor, J. 1998. "The Meaning of Research: Kids as Subjects and Kids as Inquirers." *Qualitative Inquiry* 4.3: 369–88.

Nespor, J. 1997. *Tangled Up in School: Politics, Space, Bodies, and Signs in the Educational Process.* Mahwah, NJ: Erlbaum

Nestle, M. 2002. *Food Politics: How the Food Industry Influences Nutrition and Health.* California Studies in Food and Culture. Berkeley: University of California Press.

Newman, K. 2000. *No Shame in My Game: The Working Poor in the Inner-City.* New York: Vintage.

Newman, K. 1999. *Fall from Grace: Downward Mobility in the Age of Affluence.* Berkeley: University of California Press.

Nichter, M. 2000. *Fat Talk: What Girls and Their Parents Say about Dieting.* Cambridge, MA: Harvard University Press.

Ochs, E., M. Shohet, B. Campos, and M. Beck. 2010. "Coming Together for Dinner: A Study of Working Families." In *Workplace Flexibility: Realigning 20th-Century Jobs to 21st-Century Workforce.* Eds. K. Christensen and B. Schneider. Ithaca, NY: Cornell University Press, pp. 57–70.

Oldenburg, R. 1989. *The Great Good Place: Cafes, Coffee Shops, Bookstores, Bars, Hair Salons, and Other Hangouts at the Heart of a Community.* New York: De Capo Press.

Olfman, S. (ed.). 2005. *Childhood Lost: How American Culture Is Failing Our Kids.* London: Praeger.

Oliver, J. E. 2005. *Fat Politics: The Real Story behind America's Obesity Epidemic.* New York: Oxford University Press.

Orfield, G., S. Eaton, and the Harvard Project on School Desegregation. 1998. *Dismantling Desegregation: The Quiet Reversal of* Brown v. Board of Education. New York: New Press.

Palladino, G. 1997. *Teenagers: An American History.* New York: Basic Books.

Patel, R. 2007. *Stuffed and Starved: The Hidden Battle for the World Food System.* New York: Melville House.

Paterson, M. 2006. *Consumption and Everyday Life.* New York: Routledge.

Pleck, E. 2004. "Who Are We and Where Do We Come From? Rituals, Families, and Identities." In *We Are What We Celebrate: Understanding Holidays and Rituals.* Eds. Amitai Etzioni and Jared Bloom. New York: NYU Press.

Pollen, M. 2013. *Cooked: A Natural History of Transformation.* New York: Penguin.

Pollen, M. 2008. *In Defense of Food: An Eater's Manifesto.* New York: Penguin.

Pollen, M. 2007. *Omnivore's Dilemma: A Natural History of Four Meals*. New York: Penguin.

Poppendieck, J. 2010. *Free for All: Fixing School Food in America*. Berkeley: University of California Press.

Poppendieck, J. 1999. *Sweet Charity: Emergency Food and the End of Entitlement*. New York: Penguin.

Poti, J., and B. Popkin. 2011. "Trends in Energy Intake among US Children by Eating Location and Food Source, 1977–2006." *Journal of the American Dietetic Association* 111.8 (August 2011).

Pottier, J. 1999. *Anthropology of Food: The Social Dynamics of Food Security*. New York: Polity.

Pudup, M. 2008. "It Takes a Garden: Cultivating Citizen-Subjects in Organized Garden Projects." *Geo-forum* 39: 1228–40.

Pugh, A. 2015. *The Tumbleweed Society: Working and Caring in an Age of Insecurity*. Oxford: Oxford University Press.

Pugh, A. 2009. *Longing and Belonging: Parents, Children, and Consumer Culture*. Berkeley: University of California Press.

Reay, D., G. Crozier, D. James, S. Hollingworth, K. Williams, F. Jamieson, and P. Beedell. 2008. "Re-invigorating Democracy? White Middle-Class Identities and Comprehensive Schooling." *Sociological Review* 56.2: 238–55.

Rios, V. 2012. *Punished: Policing the Lives of Black and Latino Boys*. New York: NYU Press.

Ritzer, G. 2005. *Enchanting a Disenchanting World: Revolutionizing the Means of Consumption*. 2nd ed. Thousand Oaks, CA: Pine Forge Press.

Robert, S., and M. Weaver Hightower. 2011. *School Food Politics: The Complex Ecology of Hunger and Feeding in Schools around the World*. New York: Peter Lang.

Rollins, B., E. Loken, J. Savage, and L. Birch. 2014. "Effects of Restriction on Children's Intake Differ by Child Temperament, Food Reinforcement, and Parents' Chronic Use of Restriction." *Appetite* 73.1: 31–39.

Rothblum, E., and S. Solovay (eds.). 2009. *The Fat Studies Reader*. New York: NYU Press.

Saguy, A. 2012. *What's Wrong with Fat?* Oxford: Oxford University Press.

Salazar, M. 2007. "Public Schools and Private Food: Mexicano Memories of Culture and Conflict in American School Cafeterias." *Food and Foodways* 15.3/4: 153–81.

Schlosser, E. 2001. *Fast-food Nation: The Dark Side of the All-American Meal*. Boston: Houghton Mifflin.

Schor, J. 2000. "Towards a New Politics of Consumption." In *The Consumer Society Reader*. Eds. Juliet B. Schor and Douglas B. Holt. New York: New Press.

Seligmann, L. 2013. *Broken Links, Enduring Ties: American Adoption across Race, Class, and Nation*. Palo Alto, CA: Stanford University Press.

Shapiro, L. 1986. *Perfection Salad: Women and Cooking at the Turn of the Century*. New York: Modern Library.

Slater, D. 1997. *Consumer Culture and Modernity*. Oxford: Polity.

Small, M. 2009. "'How Many Cases Do I Need?' On Science and the Logic of Case Selection in Field-Based Research." *Ethnography* 10.1: 5–38.

Stacey, J. 1997. *In the Name of the Family: Rethinking Family Values in the Postmodern Age.* Boston: Beacon.

Steinberg, S., and J. Kincheloe (eds.). 1997. *Kinder-Culture: The Corporate Construction of Childhood.* Boulder, CO: Westview.

Sterns, P. 2002. *Fat History: Bodies and Beauty in the Modern West.* New York: NYU Press.

Swidler, A. 1986. "Culture in Action: Symbols and Strategies." *American Sociological Review* 51.2: 273–86.

Taylor, C. 2004. *Modern Social Imaginaries.* Durham NC: Duke University Press.

Taylor, N. 2011. "Negotiating Popular Obesity Discourses in Adolescence: School Food, Personal Responsibility, and Gendered Food Consumption Behaviors." *Food, Culture, and Society: An International Journal of Multidisciplinary Research* 14.4: 587–606.

Thomas, N. 1991. *Entangled Objects: Exchange, Material Culture, and Colonialism in the Pacific.* Cambridge, MA: Harvard University Press.

Thornton, S. 1995. *Club Cultures: Music, Media, and Subcultural Capital.* Cambridge: Polity.

Thornton, S. 1994. "Moral Panic, the Media, and British Rave Culture." In *Microphone Fiends: Youth Music, Youth Culture.* Eds. A. Ross and T. Rose. New York: Routledge.

Tilton, J. 2010. *Dangerous or Endangered? Race and the Politics of Youth in Urban America.* New York: NYU Press.

Treuhaft, S., and A. Karpyn. 2012. "The Grocery Gap: Who Has Access to Healthy Food and Why It Matters." Report provided by PolicyLink and the Food Trust. http://www.policylink.org.

Tronto, J. 2013. *Caring Democracy: Markets, Equality, and Justice.* New York: NYU Press.

Troutt, D. 2014. *The Price of Paradise: The Cost of Inequality and a Vision of a More Equitable America.* New York: NYU Press.

Turner, V. 1969. *The Ritual Process: Structure and Anti-structure.* Chicago: Aldine.

Wacquant, L. 2010. "Crafting the Neoliberal State: Workfare, Prisonfare, and Social Insecurity." *Sociological Forum* 25.2: 197–220.

Wacquant, L. 2006. *Body and Soul: Notebook of an Apprentice Boxer.* Chicago: University of Chicago Press.

Warikoo, N. 2013. *Balancing Acts: Youth Culture in the Global City.* Berkeley: University of California Press.

Watson J., and M. Caldwell (eds.). 2005. *The Cultural Politics of Food and Eating: A Reader.* Oxford: Blackwell.

Weaver-Hightower, M. 2011. "Why Education Researchers Should Take School Food Seriously." *Education Research* 40.1: 15–21.

Weis, L. 1990. *Working Class without Work: High School Students in a De-Industrialized Economy.* New York: Routledge.

Wells, J. 2012. "Obesity as Malnutrition: The Role of Capitalism in the Obesity Global Epidemic." *American Journal of Human Biology* 24: 261–76.

Willard, M., and J. Austin. 1998. *Generations of Youth: Youth Cultures and History in Twentieth-Century America*. New York: NYU Press.

Wilk, R. 2008. "'Real Belizean Food': Building Local Identity in the Transnational Caribbean." In *Food and Culture: A Reader*. 2nd ed. Eds. Carole Counihan and Penny Van Esterik. New York: Routledge.

Wilkins, A. 2008. *Wannabes, Goths, and Christians: The Boundaries of Sex, Style, and Status*. Chicago: University of Chicago Press.

Williams, P. 1992. *Alchemy of Race and Rights: The Diary of a Law Professor*. Cambridge, MA: Harvard University Press.

Willis, P. 1990. "Everyday Life and Symbolic Creativity." *Common Culture: Symbolic Work at Play in the Everyday Cultures of the Young*. Boulder, CO: Westview.

Willis, P. 1977. *Learning to Labour*. Aldershot: Saxon House.

Winne, M. 2008. *Closing the Food Gap: Resetting the Table in the Land of Plenty*. Boston: Beacon.

Winson, A. 2013. *The Industrial Diet: The Degradation of Food and the Struggle for Eating*. New York: NYU Press.

Yan, Y. 2005. "Of Hamburger and Social Space: Consuming McDonald's in Beijing." In *The Cultural Politics of Food and Eating*. Eds. J. Watson and M. Caldwell. London: Blackwell.

Zelizer, V. 2005. *The Purchase of Intimacy*. Princeton, NJ: Princeton University Press.

Zelizer, V. 1997. *The Social Meaning of Money: Pin Money, Paychecks, Poor Relief, and Other Currency*. Princeton, NJ: Princeton University Press.

Zelizer, V. 1985. *Pricing the Priceless Child: The Changing Social Value of Children*. New York: Basic Books.

Zerubavel, E. 1991. *The Fine Line: Making Distinctions in Everyday Life*. Chicago: University of Chicago Press.

Zukin, S. 2003. *Point of Purchase: How Shopping Changed American Culture*. New York: Routledge.

INDEX

academics, 92–93

accessibility: in ethnography, 177; as justice issue, 165; of McDonald's, 129–32; for poverty, 165

achievement gap, 82–84, 207n21; race in, 83

administrative staff: at cafeteria, 85–86; in conflict play, 89; recognition from, 86; with students, 85–86

adolescent boys, 11

adolescent girls: body consciousness of, 9; food relationships of, 8–9; health discourse of, 9

adults, 3; on agenda, 179–80; anxiety of, 153–57; authority of, 135–36; as informants, 178; interviews with, 183–84; at McDonald's, 135; researcher as, 176–77; in youth research, 179–81. *See also* parents

Advanced Placement (AP) courses, 82–83

advertising, 18

African Americans, 59. *See also* black Americans

age: in critical youth studies, 171; social meaning and, 11–12; in studying youth, 176

agenda, 179–80

American Community Survey, 34, 161

anxiety: of adults, 153–57; of childhood obesity, 154; in modernity, 155–56

AP. *See* Advanced Placement

Appadurai, Arun, 5

"Appetite as Voice" (Brumberg), 188n2

Arby's, 150–51

Arcadia Center for Sustainable Food and Agriculture, 184

authority: of adults, 135–36; as researcher, 176–77

bartering, 100–101, 118–20, 138. *See also* gift economy

Barthes, Roland, 81

Baskin-Robbins, 1

bathrooms, 205n3

belonging, 155; connection to, 161; in family food memory narratives, 42–43; symbolic importance of, 51

Berensin, Anna, 115, 125

Besen-Cassino, Yasemin, 187n1

Bettie, Julie, 92

Big Mac rap, 123

Biltekoff, Charlotte, 14

Binkley, Sam, 156

bio-bullying, 15

biology, 171; predetermined desire in, 11

biopolitics, 14

birthday cakes, 13

black Americans: in cafeteria, 5, 54, 58–59, 79, 83–86, 91–92, 132–33; in McDonald's, 130; youth space of, 81

BMI. *See* Body Mass Index

body: boundaries and play, 88–89; play of, 143–44

body consciousness: of adolescent girls, 9; as feminine concern, 8–9, 96

Body Mass Index (BMI) calculation, 190n47

boredom, 120, 121; commercial foods as break in, 117

ABOUT THE AUTHOR

Amy L. Best is Professor of Sociology in the Department of Sociology and Anthropology at George Mason University. She is author of *Prom Night: Youth, Schools, and Popular Culture*, which was selected for a 2002 American Educational Studies Association Critics' Choice Award, and of *Fast Cars, Cool Rides: The Accelerating World of Youth and Their Cars*.